Provided as a service to oncology
by Lederle Laboratories

UICC International Union Against Cancer

TNM

Classification of Malignant Tumours

Edited by P. Hermanek and L. H. Sobin

Fourth, Fully Revised Edition

Springer-Verlag Berlin Heidelberg New York
London Paris Tokyo 1987

UICC
3, rue du Conseil-Général
CH-1205 Geneva, Switzerland

Editors:

Prof. Dr. P. Hermanek
Abteilung für Klinische Pathologie
Chirurgische Universitätsklinik Erlangen-Nürnberg
Maximiliansplatz
D-8520 Erlangen, Federal Republic of Germany

L. H. Sobin, M. D.
Department of Gastrointestinal Pathology
Armed Forces Institute of Pathology
Washington, D. C. 20306, USA

All previous English editions were published by the UICC 1968, 1974, 1978

ISBN 3-540-17366-8 Springer-Verlag Berlin Heidelberg New York
ISBN 0-387-17366-8 Springer-Verlag New York Berlin Heidelberg

Library of Congress Cataloging in Publication Data
TNM classification of malignant tumours.
1. Tumors-Classification. I. Hermanek, P. (Paul) II. Sobin, L. H. III. International Union
against Cancer.
RC258. T583 1987   616.99'4'0021   87-4695   ISBN 0-387-17366-8 (U.S.)

Typesetting and Bookbinding: Appl, Wemding. Printing: aprinta, Wemding
2121/3145-54321

They are called wise
who put things in their right order

Thomas Aquinas

Acknowledgements

The Editors have much pleasure in acknowledging the great help received from the members of the TNM Committee and the national and international organizations listed on pp. XV to XVIII.

The fourth edition of the TNM Classification is the result of many unification and editorial meetings. The production of this edition would not have been possible without the organization of the meetings by the AJCC and the Geneva office of the UICC. Gratitude should also be expressed to Mrs. Judith Wagner, Erlangen, Federal Republic of Germany, who has so competently and patiently transformed the handwritten sheets and numerous corrections into an orderly typescript.

Support of the TNM Project by the National Cancer Institute (USA) through grants CA 05096 and CA 38193 is gratefully acknowledged.

Table of Contents

Contents

Abbreviations

c	clinical, p. 5
C	certainty factor, p. 10
G	histopathological grading
ICD-O	International Classification of Diseases for Oncology
ICD-O M	morphology rubric of ICD-O
ICD-O T	topography rubric of ICD-O
m	multiple tumours, p. 6
M	distant metastasis
N	regional lymph node metastasis
p	pathological, p. 5
r	recurrent tumour, p. 9
R	residual tumour after treatment, p. 10
T	extent of primary tumour
y	classification after initial multimodal therapy, p. 9

National Committees and International Organizations

AJCC	The American Joint Committee on Cancer
BIJC	The British Isles Joint TNM Classification Committee
CNC	The Canadian National TNM Committee
CNU-TNM	Comité Nacional Uruguayo TNM
DSK	Deutschsprachiges TNM-Komitee
EORTC	The European Organization for Research on Treatment of Cancer
FIGO	Fédération Internationale de Gynécologie et d'Obstétrique
FTNM	The French TNM Group
ICC	The Italian Committee for TNM Cancer Classification
JJC	The Japanese Joint Committee
SIOP	La Société Internationale d'Oncologie Pédiatrique

Members of the UICC Committees Associated With the TNM System

In 1950 the UICC appointed a *Committee on Tumour Nomenclature and Statistics*. In 1954 this Committee became known as the *Committee on Clinical Stage Classification and Applied Statistics* and since 1966 it has been the *Committee on TNM Classification*. The members who have served on these committees are as follows:

Anderson, W. A. D.	USA
Baclesse, F.	France
Badellino, F.	Italy
Barajas-Vallejo, E.	Mexico
Blinov, N.	USSR
Bucalossi, P.	Italy
Burn, I.	United Kingdom
Bush, R. S.	Canada
Carr, D. T.	USA
Copeland, M. M.	USA
Costachel, O.	Romania
Denoix, P.	France
Fischer, A. W.	Federal Republic of Germany
Gentil, F.	Brazil
Ginsberg, R.	Canada
Hamperl, H.	Federal Republic of Germany
Harmer, M. H.	United Kingdom
Hayat, M.	France
Hermanek, P.	Federal Republic of Germany
Hultberg, S.	Sweden
Hutter, R. V. P.	USA
Ichikawa, H.	Japan

INTRODUCTION

The History of the TNM System

The TNM System for the classification of malignant tumours was developed by Pierre Denoix (France) between the years 1943 and 1952.[1]

In 1950 the UICC appointed a *Committee on Tumour Nomenclature and Statistics* and adopted, as a basis for its work on clinical stage classification, the general definitions of local extension of malignant tumours suggested by the World Health Organization (WHO) Sub-Committee on The Registration of Cases of Cancer as well as their Statistical Presentation.[2]

In 1953 the Committee held a joint meeting with the International Commission on Stage-Grouping in Cancer and Presentation of the Results of Treatment of Cancer appointed by the International Congress of Radiology. Agreement was reached on a general technique for classification by anatomical extent of disease, using the TNM system.

In 1954 the Research Commission of the UICC set up a special *Committee on Clinical Stage Classification and Applied Statistics* to "pursue studies in this field and to extend the general technique of classification to cancer at all sites".

In 1958 the Committee published its first recommendations for the clinical stage classification of cancers of the breast and

---

[1] Denoix, P. F.: Bull. Inst. Nat. Hyg. (Paris) 1: 1–69 (1944) and 5: 52–82 (1944).
[2] World Health Organization Technical Report Series, no. 53, July 1952, pp. 47–48.

larynx and for the presentation of results.[3] A second publication in 1959 presented revised proposals for the breast, for clinical use and evaluation over a 5-year period (1960–1964).[4]

Between 1960 and 1967 the Committee published nine brochures describing proposals for the classification of 23 sites. It was recommended that the classification proposals for each site be subjected to prospective or retrospective trial for a 5-year period.

In 1968 these brochures were combined in a booklet, the *Livre de Poche* and a year later, a complementary booklet was published detailing recommendations for the setting-up of field trials, for the presentation of end results and for the determination and expression of cancer survival rates. The *Livre de Poche* was subsequently translated into 11 languages.

In 1974 and 1978, second and third editions were published containing new site classifications and amendments to previously published classifications. The third edition was enlarged and revised in 1982. It contained new classifications for selected tumours of childhood. This was carried out in collaboration with La Société Internationale d'Oncologie Pédiatrique (SIOP). A classification of ophthalmic tumours was published separately in 1985.

Over the years some users introduced variations in the rules of classification of certain sites. In order to correct this development, the antithesis of standardization, the national TNM committees in 1982 agreed to formulate a single TNM. A series of meetings was held to unify and update existing classifications as well as to develop new ones. The result is the present fourth edition of the TNM. The rules of classification and stage grouping correspond exactly with those appearing in the third edition of the *AJCC Manual for Staging of Cancer* (1987) and have the

---

[3] International Union Against Cancer (UICC), Committee on Clinical Stage Classification and Applied Statistics: Clinical stage classification and presentation of results, malignant tumours of the breast and larynx. Paris, 1958.

[4] International Union Against Cancer (UICC), Committee on Stage Classification and Applied Statistics: Clinical stage classification and presentation of results, malignant tumours of the breast. Paris, 1959.

approval of all national TNM committees. These are listed on pages XV–XVIII together with the names of members of the UICC committees who have been associated with the TNM system.

The UICC recognizes the need for stability in the TNM classification so that data can be accumulated in an orderly way over reasonable periods of time. Accordingly, it is the intention that the classifications published in this booklet should remain unchanged until some major advances in diagnosis or treatment, relevant to a particular site, require reconsideration of the current classification.

To develop and sustain a classification system acceptable to all requires the closest liaison by all national and international committees. Only in this way will all oncologists be able to use a "common language" in comparing their clinical material and in assessing the results of treatment. The continuing objective of the UICC is to achieve common consent in a classification of the anatomical extent of disease.

The Principles of the TNM System

The practice of dividing cancer cases into groups according to so-called stages arose from the fact that survival rates were higher for cases in which the disease was localized than for those in which the disease had extended beyond the organ of origin. These groups were often referred to as early cases and late cases, implying some regular progression with time. Actually, the stage of disease at the time of diagnosis may be a reflection not only of the rate of growth and extension of the neoplasm but also of the type of tumour and of the tumour-host relationship.

The staging of cancer is hallowed by tradition and for the purpose of analysis of groups of patients it is often necessary to use such a method. The UICC believes that it is preferable to reach agreement on the recording of accurate information on the extent of the disease for each site, because the precise clinical description and histopathological classification (when possible) of malignant neoplasms may serve a number of related objectives, namely to

1. Aid the clinician in the planning of treatment
2. Give some indication of prognosis
3. Assist in evaluation of the results of treatment
4. Facilitate the exchange of information between treatment centres
5. Contribute to the continuing investigation of human cancer.

The principal purpose to be served by international agreement on the classification of cancer cases by extent of disease is to provide a method of conveying clinical experience to others without ambiguity.

There are many bases or axes of classification, for example the anatomical site and the clinical and pathological extent of disease, the reported duration of symptoms or signs, the sex and age of the patient, and the histological type and grade. All of these bases or axes represent variables which are known to have an influence on the outcome of the disease. Classification by anatomical extent of disease as determined clinically and histopathologically (when possible) is the one with which the TNM system primarily deals.

The clinician's immediate task is to make a judgment as to prognosis and a decision as to the most effective course of treatment. This judgment and this decision require, among other things, an objective assessment of the anatomical extent of the disease. In accomplishing this, the trend is away from "staging" to meaningful description, with or without some form of summarization.

To meet the stated objectives we need a system of classification
1. Whose basic principles are applicable to all sites regardless of treatment
2. Which may be supplemented later by information which becomes available from histopathology and/or surgery.

The TNM system meets these requirements.

The General Rules of the TNM System

The TNM system for describing the anatomical extent of disease
is based on the assessment of three components:

T – The extent of the primary tumour

N – The absence or presence and extent of regional lymph node
metastasis

M – The absence or presence of distant metastasis.

The addition of numbers to these three components indicates the
extent of the malignant disease, thus:

T0, T1, T2, T3, T4   N0, N1, N2, N3   M0, M1

In effect the system is a "shorthand notation" for describing
the extent of a particular malignant tumour.

The general rules applicable to all sites are as follows:

1. All cases should be confirmed microscopically. Any cases not
   so proved must be reported separately.
2. Two classifications are described for each site, namely:
   a) *Clinical classification* (Pre-treatment clinical classification),
      designated **TNM** (or cTNM). This is based on evidence
      acquired before treatment. Such evidence arises from phys-
      ical examination, imaging, endoscopy, biopsy, surgical
      exploration and other relevant examinations.
   b) *Pathological classification* (Post-surgical histopathological
      classification), designated **pTNM.** This is based on the evi-
      dence acquired before treatment, supplemented or modi-
      fied by the additional evidence acquired from surgery and
      from pathological examination. The pathological assess-
      ment of the primary tumour (pT)[5] entails a resection of the
      primary tumour or biopsy adequate to evaluate the highest
      pT category. The pathological assessment of the regional
      lymph nodes (pN) entails removal of nodes adequate to
      validate the absence of regional lymph node metastasis

---

[5] Substantial changes in the 4th edition compared to the previous one are
marked by a thick line at the left-hand side of the page. The same is true for
the new classifications of previously unclassified tumours.

(pN0) and sufficient to evaluate the highest pN category. The pathological assessment of distant metastasis (pM) entails microscopic examination.

3. After assigning T, N and M and/or pT, pN and pM categories, these may be grouped into stages. The TNM classification and stage grouping, once established, must remain unchanged in the medical records. The clinical stage is essential to select and evaluate therapy, while the pathological stage provides the most precise data to estimate prognosis and calculate end results.

4. If there is doubt concerning the correct T, N or M category to which a particular case should be allotted, then the lower (i.e. less advanced) category should be chosen. This will also be reflected in the stage grouping.

5. In the case of multiple simultaneous tumours in one organ, the tumour with the highest T category should be classified and the multiplicity or the number of tumours should be indicated in parentheses, e.g. T2 (m) or T2 (5). In simultaneous bilateral cancers of paired organs, each tumour should be classified independently. In tumours of the thyroid and liver, nephroblastoma and neuroblastoma, multiplicity is a criterion of T classification.

The Anatomical Regions and Sites

The sites in this classification are listed by code number of the International Classification of Diseases for Oncology (ICD-O, World Health Organization, 1976).

Each region or site is described under the following headings:
Rules for classification with the procedures for assessing the T, N and M categories
Anatomical sites, and subsites if appropriate
Definition of the regional lymph nodes
TNM Clinical classification
pTNM Pathological classification
Stage grouping
Summary for the region or site

TNM Clinical Classification

The following general definitions are used throughout:

T – Primary Tumour

TX   Primary tumour cannot be assessed
T0   No evidence of primary tumour
Tis   Carcinoma in situ
T1, T2, T3, T4   Increasing size and/or local extent of the primary tumour

N – Regional Lymph Nodes

NX   Regional lymph nodes cannot be assessed
N0   No regional lymph node metastasis
N1, N2, N3   Increasing involvement of regional lymph nodes

Notes: Direct extension of the primary tumour into lymph nodes is classified as lymph node metastasis.

Metastasis in any lymph node other than regional is classified as a distant metastasis.

M – Distant Metastasis

MX   Presence of distant metastasis cannot be assessed
M0   No distant metastasis
M1   Distant metastasis

The category M1 may be further specified according to the following notation:

Pulmonary	PUL	Bone marrow	MAR
Osseous	OSS	Pleura	PLE
Hepatic	HEP	Peritoneum	PER
Brain	BRA	Skin	SKI
Lymph nodes	LYM	Other	OTH

Subdivisions of TNM

Subdivisions of some main categories are available for those who need greater specificity (e. g. T1a, 1b or N2a, 2b).

pTNM Pathological Classification

The following general definitions are used throughout:

pT – Primary Tumour

pTX Primary tumour cannot be assessed histologically
pT0   No histological evidence of primary tumour
pTis Carcinoma in situ
pT1, pT2, pT3, pT4   Increasing extent of the primary tumour
        histologically

pN – Regional Lymph Nodes

pNX Regional lymph nodes cannot be assessed histologically
pN0   No regional lymph node metastasis histologically
pN1, pN2, pN3   Increasing involvement of regional lymph
        nodes histologically

Notes: Direct extension of the primary tumour into lymph nodes is classified
        as lymph node metastasis.
        When size is a criterion for pN classification, e. g. in breast carci-
        noma, measurement is made of the metastasis not of the entire lymph
        node.

pM – Distant Metastasis

pMX Presence of distant metastasis cannot be assessed micro-
        scopically
pM0   No distant metastasis microscopically
pM1   Distant metastasis microscopically
The category pM1 may be further specified in the same way as
M1 (see p. 7).

Subdivisions of pTNM

Subdivisions of some main categories are available for those who need greater specificity (e.g. pT1a, 1b or pN2a, 2b).

Histopathological Grading

In most sites further information regarding the primary tumour may be recorded under the following heading:

G - Histopathological Grading

GX   Grade of differentiation cannot be assessed
G1   Well differentiated
G2   Moderately differentiated
G3   Poorly differentiated
G4   Undifferentiated

Additional Descriptors

The use of the following descriptors is optional.

y Symbol

In those cases in which classification is performed during or following initial multimodal therapy, the TNM or pTNM categories are identified by a "y" prefix (e.g. yT2N1M0 or ypT2pN2pM0).

r Symbol

Recurrent tumours are identified by the prefix "r" (e.g. rT2N0M0 or rpT3pN1pMX).

C-Factor

The C-factor, or certainty factor, reflects the validity of classification according to the diagnostic methods employed. Its use is optional.

The C-factor definitions are:

C1   Evidence from standard diagnostic means (e. g. inspection, palpation and standard radiography, intraluminal endoscopy for tumours of certain organs)

C2   Evidence obtained by special diagnostic means (e. g. radiographic imaging in special projections, tomography, computerized tomography [CT], ultrasonography, lymphography, angiography; scintigraphy; magnetic resonance imaging [MRI]; endoscopy, biopsy, and cytology)

C3   Evidence from surgical exploration, including biopsy and cytology

C4   Evidence of the extent of disease following definitive surgery and pathological examination of the resected specimen

C5   Evidence from autopsy

Example: Degrees of C may be applied to the T, N and M categories. A case might be described as T3C2, N2C1, M0C2.

The TNM clinical classification is therefore equivalent to C1, C2 and C3 in varying degrees of certainty, while the pTNM pathological classification is equivalent to C4.

Residual Tumour (R) Classification

The absence or presence of residual tumour after treatment is described by the symbol R. Its use is optional.

RX   Presence of residual tumour cannot be assessed

R0   No residual tumour

R1   Microscopic residual tumour

R2   Macroscopic residual tumour

Stage Grouping

Classification by the TNM system achieves reasonably precise description and recording of the apparent anatomical extent of disease. A tumour with four degrees of T, three degrees of N, and two degrees of M will have 24 TNM categories. For purposes of tabulation and analysis, except in very large series, it is necessary to condense these categories into a convenient number of TNM stage groups.

Carcinoma in situ is categorized stage 0, cases with distant metastasis stage IV.

The grouping adopted is such as to ensure, as far as possible, that each group is more or less homogeneous in respect of survival, and that the survival rates of these groups for each cancer site are distinctive.

Site Summary

As an aide-mémoire or as a means of reference, a simple summary of the chief points which distinguish the most important categories is added at the end of each site. These abridged definitions are not, and do not pretend to be, completely adequate and the full definitions should always be consulted.

Related Classifications

Since 1958 the WHO has been involved in a programme aimed at providing internationally acceptable criteria for the histological diagnosis of tumours. This has resulted in the *International Histological Classification of Tumours* which contains, in an illustrated 25-volume series, definitions of tumour types and a proposed nomenclature.

The *WHO International Classification of Diseases for Oncology (ICD-O)* was developed as a coding system for neoplasms by topography and morphology and for indicating behaviour (e.g.

malignant, benign). This coded nomenclature is identical in the morphology field for neoplasms to the *Systematized Nomenclature of Medicine* (SNOMED) published by the College of American Pathologists in 1976.

In the interest of promoting national and international collaboration in cancer research and specifically of facilitating co-operation in clinical investigations, it is recommended that the *International Histological Classification of Tumours* be used for classification and definition of tumour types and that the ICD-O code be used for storage and retrieval of data.

Substantial changes in the 4th edition compared to the previous one are marked by a thick line at the left-hand side of the page. The same is true for new classifications of previously unclassified tumours.

HEAD AND NECK TUMOURS

Introductory Notes

The following sites are included:

Lip, Oral cavity	Maxillary sinus
Pharynx	Salivary glands
Larynx	Thyroid gland

Each site is described under the following headings:
Rules for classification with the procedures for assessing the T, N and M categories. Additional methods may be used when they enhance the accuracy of appraisal before treatment
Anatomical sites and subsites where appropriate
Definition of the regional lymph nodes
TNM Clinical classification
pTNM Pathological classification
G Histopathological grading
Stage grouping
Summary

Additional Descriptors

When appropriate, the y symbol, the r symbol and the C-factor category may be added (see p. 9).

Regional Lymph Nodes

The definitions of the N categories for all head and neck sites except thyroid gland are:

N – Regional Lymph Nodes

NX   Regional lymph nodes cannot be assessed
N0   No regional lymph node metastasis
N1   Metastasis in a single ipsilateral lymph node, 3 cm or less in greatest dimension
N2   Metastasis in a single ipsilateral lymph node, more than 3 cm but not more than 6 cm in greatest dimension, or in multiple ipsilateral lymph nodes, none more than 6 cm in greatest dimension, or in bilateral or contralateral lymph nodes, none more than 6 cm in greatest dimension
    N2a   Metastasis in a single ipsilateral lymph node, more than 3 cm but not more than 6 cm in greatest dimension
    N2b   Metastasis in multiple ipsilateral lymph nodes, none more than 6 cm in greatest dimension
    N2c   Metastasis in bilateral or contralateral lymph nodes, none more than 6 cm in greatest dimension
N3   Metastasis in a lymph node more than 6 cm in greatest dimension

Distant Metastasis

The definitions of the M categories for all head and neck sites are:

M – Distant Metastasis

MX   Presence of distant metastasis cannot be assessed
M0   No distant metastasis
M1   Distant metastasis

The category M1 may be further specified according to the following notation:

Pulmonary	PUL	Bone marrow	MAR
Osseous	OSS	Pleura	PLE
Hepatic	HEP	Peritoneum	PER
Brain	BRA	Skin	SKI
Lymph nodes	LYM	Other	OTH

Histopathological Grading

The definitions of the G categories apply to all head and neck sites. These are:

G – Histopathological Grading

GX   Grade of differentiation cannot be assessed
G1   Well differentiated
G2   Moderately differentiated
G3   Poorly differentiated
G4   Undifferentiated

R Classification

The absence or presence of residual tumour after treatment may be described by the symbol R. The definitions of the R classification apply to all head and neck sites. These are:

RX   Presence of residual tumour cannot be assessed
R0   No residual tumour
R1   Microscopic residual tumour
R2   Macroscopic residual tumour

Lip and Oral Cavity (ICD-O 140, 141, 143–145)

Rules for Classification

The classification applies only to squamous-cell carcinoma of the vermilion surfaces of the lips and to carcinoma of the oral cavity. There should be histological confirmation of the disease.

The following are the procedures for assessment of the T, N and M categories:

T categories	Physical examination and imaging
N categories	Physical examination and imaging
M categories	Physical examination and imaging

Anatomical Sites and Subsites

Lip

1. Upper lip, vermilion surface (140.0)
2. Lower lip, vermilion surface (140.1)
3. Commissures (140.6)

Oral Cavity

1. Buccal mucosa
   i) Mucosal surfaces of upper and lower lips (140.3, 4)
   ii) Mucosal surface of cheeks (145.0)
   iii) Retromolar areas (145.6)
   iv) Bucco-alveolar sulci, upper and lower (145.1)
2. Upper alveolus and gingiva (143.0)
3. Lower alveolus and gingiva (143.1)
4. Hard palate (145.2)
5. Tongue
   i) Dorsal surface and lateral borders anterior to vallate papillae (anterior two-thirds) (141.1,2)
   ii) Inferior surface (141.3)
6. Floor of mouth (144)

Regional Lymph Nodes

The regional lymph nodes are the cervical nodes.

TNM Clinical Classification

T – Primary Tumour

TX   Primary tumour cannot be assessed
T0   No evidence of primary tumour
Tis   Carcinoma in situ

T1   Tumour 2 cm or less in greatest dimension
T2   Tumour more than 2 cm but not more than 4 cm in greatest dimension
T3   Tumour more than 4 cm in greatest dimension
T4   *Lip:* Tumour invades adjacent structures, e.g. through cortical bone, tongue, skin of neck
       Oral Cavity: Tumour invades adjacent structures, e.g. through cortical bone, into deep (extrinsic) muscle of tongue, maxillary sinus, skin

N – Regional Lymph Nodes

See definitions p.14.

M – Distant Metastasis

See definitions p.14.

pTNM Pathological Classification

The pT, pN and pM categories correspond to the T, N and M categories.

G Histopathological Grading

See definitions p. 15.

Stage Grouping

Stage 0	Tis	N0	M0
Stage I	T1	N0	M0
Stage II	T2	N0	M0
Stage III	T3	N0	M0
	T1	N1	M0
	T2	N1	M0
	T3	N1	M0
Stage IV	T4	N0, N1	M0
	Any T	N2, N3	M0
	Any T	Any N	M1

Summary

Lip, Oral Cavity	
T1	≤ 2 cm
T2	> 2 to 4 cm
T3	> 4 cm
T4	Adjacent structures
N1	Ipsilateral single ≤ 3 cm
N2	Ipsilateral single > 3 to 6 cm
	Ipsilateral multiple ≤ 6 cm
	Bilateral, contralateral ≤ 6 cm
N3	> 6 cm

Pharynx (ICD-O 141.0, 154.3,4, 146–148)

Rules for Classification

The classification applies only to carcinoma. There should be histological confirmation of the disease.

The following are the procedures for assessment of the T, N and M categories:

T categories   Physical examination, endoscopy and imaging
N categories   Physical examination and imaging
M categories   Physical examination and imaging

Anatomical Sites and Subsites

Oropharynx (141.0, 145.3,4, 146)

1. Anterior wall (glosso-epiglottic area)
    i)   Tongue posterior to the vallate papillae (base of tongue or posterior third) (141.0)
    ii)   Vallecula (146.3)
2. Lateral wall (146.6)
    i)   Tonsil (146.0)
    ii)   Tonsillar fossa (146.1) and faucial pillars (146.2)
    iii) Glossotonsillar sulci (146.2)
3. Posterior wall (146.7)
4. Superior wall
    i)   Inferior surface of soft palate (145.3)
    ii)   Uvula (145.4)

Nasopharynx (147)

1. Posterosuperior wall: extends from the level of the junction of the hard and soft palates to the base of the skull (147.0,1)

2. Lateral wall: including the fossa of Rosenmüller (147.2)
3. Inferior wall: consists of the superior surface of the soft palate (147.3)

Note: The margin of the choanal orifices, including the posterior margin of the nasal septum, is included with the nasal fossa.

Hypopharynx (148)

1. Pharyngo-oesophageal junction (postcricoid area) (148.0): extends from the level of the arytenoid cartilages and connecting folds to the inferior border of the cricoid cartilage
2. Pyriform sinus (148.1): extends from the pharyngo-epiglottic fold to the upper end of the oesophagus. It is bounded laterally by the thyroid cartilage and medially by the surface of the aryepiglottic fold (148.2) and the arytenoid and cricoid cartilages.
3. Posterior pharyngeal wall (148.3): extends from the level of the floor of the vallecula to the level of the crico-arytenoid joints

Regional Lymph Nodes

The regional lymph nodes are the cervical nodes.

TNM Clinical Classification

T – Primary Tumour

TX   Primary tumour cannot be assessed
T0   No evidence of primary tumour
Tis   Carcinoma in situ

Oropharynx

T1   Tumour 2 cm or less in greatest dimension
T2   Tumour more than 2 cm but not more than 4 cm in greatest
      . dimension
T3   Tumour more than 4 cm in greatest dimension

T4   Tumour invades adjacent structures, e.g. through cortical
      bone, soft tissues of neck, deep (extrinsic) muscle of
      tongue

Nasopharynx

T1   Tumour limited to one subsite of nasopharynx (see p. 19)
T2   Tumour invades more than one subsite of nasopharynx
T3   Tumour invades nasal cavity and/or oropharynx
T4   Tumour invades skull and/or cranial nerve(s)

Hypopharynx

T1   Tumour limited to one subsite of hypopharynx (see p. 20)
T2   Tumour invades more than one subsite of hypopharynx or
      an adjacent site, *without* fixation of hemilarynx
T3   Tumour invades more than one subsite of hypopharynx or
      an adjacent site, *with* fixation of hemilarynx
T4   Tumour invades adjacent structures, e.g. cartilage or soft
      tissues of neck

N – Regional Lymph Nodes

See definitions p. 14.

M – Distant Metastasis

See definitions p. 14.

pTNM Pathological Classification

The pT, pN and pM categories correspond to the T, N and M
categories.

G Histopathological Grading

See definitions p. 15.

Stage Grouping

Stage 0	Tis	N0	M0
Stage I	T1	N0	M0
Stage II	T2	N0	M0
Stage III	T3	N0	M0
	T1	N1	M0
	T2	N1	M0
	T3	N1	M0
Stage IV	T4	N0, N1	M0
	Any T	N2, N3	M0
	Any T	Any N	M1

Summary

Pharynx	
	Oropharynx
T1	≤ 2 cm
T2	> 2 to 4 cm
T3	> 4 cm
T4	Invades bone, muscle etc.
	Nasopharynx
T1	One subsite
T2	> One subsite
T3	Invades nose/oropharynx
T4	Invades skull/cranial nerve
	Hypopharynx
T1	One subsite
T2	> One subsite or adjacent site, without larynx fixation
T3	With larynx fixation
T4	Invades cartilage, neck etc.
	All Sites
N1	Ipsilateral single ≤ 3 cm
N2	Ipsilateral single > 3 to 6 cm
	Ipsilateral multiple ≤ 6 cm
	Bilateral, contralateral ≤ 6 cm
N3	> 6 cm

Larynx (ICD-O 161)

Rules for Classification

The classification applies only to carcinoma. There should be histological confirmation of the disease.

The following are the procedures for assessment of the T, N and M categories:

T categories Physical examination, laryngoscopy and imaging
N categories Physical examination and imaging
M categories Physical examination and imaging

Anatomical Sites and Subsites

1. Supraglottis (161.1)
   Epilarynx (including marginal zone)
   i)   Suprahyoid epiglottis (including the tip)
   ii) Aryepiglottic fold
   iii) Arytenoid
   Supraglottis excluding epilarynx
   iv) Infrahyoid epiglottis
   v)   Ventricular bands (false cords)
   vi) Ventricular cavities
2. Glottis (161.0)
   i)   Vocal cords
   ii) Anterior commissure
   iii) Posterior commissure
3. Subglottis (161.2)

Regional Lymph Nodes

The regional lymph nodes are the cervical nodes.

TNM Clinical Classification

T – Primary Tumour

TX   Primary tumour cannot be assessed
T0   No evidence of primary tumour
Tis   Carcinoma in situ

Supraglottis

T1   Tumour limited to one subsite of supraglottis (see p. 23), with normal vocal cord mobility
T2   Tumour invades more than one subsite of supraglottis or glottis, with normal vocal cord mobility
T3   Tumour limited to larynx with vocal cord fixation and/or invades postcricoid area, medial wall of piriform sinus or pre-epiglottic tissues
T4   Tumour invades through thyroid cartilage and/or extends to other tissues beyond the larynx, e.g. to oropharynx, soft tissues of neck

Glottis

T1   Tumour limited to vocal cord(s) (may involve anterior or posterior commissures) with normal mobility
    T1a   Tumour limited to one vocal cord
    T1b   Tumour involves both vocal cords
T2   Tumour extends to supraglottis and/or subglottis, and/or with impaired vocal cord mobility
T3   Tumour limited to the larynx with vocal cord fixation
T4   Tumour invades through thyroid cartilage and/or extends to other tissues beyond the larynx, e.g. to oropharynx, soft tissues of the neck

Subglottis

T1   Tumour limited to the subglottis
T2   Tumour extends to vocal cord(s) with normal or impaired mobility

T3   Tumour limited to the larynx with vocal cord fixation
T4   Tumour invades through cricoid or thyroid cartilage and/
      or extends to other tissues beyond the larynx, e.g. to oro-
      pharynx, soft tissues of the neck

N – Regional Lymph Nodes

See definitions p.14.

M – Distant Metastasis

See definitions p.14.

pTNM Pathological Classification

The pT, pN and pM categories correspond to the T, N and M
categories.

G Histopathological Grading

See definitions p.15.

Stage Grouping

Stage 0	Tis	N0	M0
Stage I	T1	N0	M0
Stage II	T2	N0	M0
Stage III	T3	N0	M0
	T1	N1	M0
	T2	N1	M0
	T3	N1	M0
Stage IV	T4	N0, N1	M0
	Any T	N2, N3	M0
	Any T	Any N	M1

Summary

Larynx		
		Glottis
T1		Limited/mobile
	T1a	One cord
	T1b	Both cords
T2		Extends to supra- or subglottis/impaired mobility
T3		Cord fixation
T4		Extends beyond larynx
		Supra- and Subglottis
T1		Limited/mobile
T2		Extends to glottis/mobile
T3		Cord fixation
T4		Extends beyond larynx
		All Regions
N1		Ipsilateral single $\leqslant 3$ cm
N2		Ipsilateral single > 3 to 6 cm
		Ipsilateral multiple $\leqslant 6$ cm
		Bilateral, contralateral $\leqslant 6$ cm
N3		> 6 cm

Maxillary Sinus (ICD-O 160.2)

Rules for Classification

The classification applies only to carcinoma. There should be histological confirmation of the disease.

The following are the procedures for assessment of the T, N and M categories:

T categories   Physical examination and imaging
N categories   Physical examination and imaging
M categories   Physical examination and imaging

Anatomical Division

Ohngren's Line is defined as the plane passing through the inner canthus and the mandibular angle and which divides the upper jaw into the superoposterior structure *(suprastructure)* and infero-anterior structure *(infrastructure)*. The suprastructure includes the posterior bony wall and posterior half of the superior bony wall. The other bony walls belong to the infrastructure.

Regional Lymph Nodes

The Regional Lymph Nodes are the cervical nodes.

TNM Clinical Classification

T - Primary Tumour

TX   Primary tumour cannot be assessed
T0   No evidence of primary tumour
Tis   Carcinoma in situ

T1   Tumour limited to the antral mucosa with no erosion or destruction of bone
T2   Tumour with erosion or destruction of the infrastructure (see anatomical division above) including the hard palate and/or the middle nasal meatus
T3   Tumour invades any of the following: skin of cheek, posterior wall of the maxillary sinus, floor or medial wall of orbit, anterior ethmoid sinus
T4   Tumour invades the orbital contents and/or any of the following: cribriform plate, posterior ethmoid or sphenoid sinuses, nasopharynx, soft palate, pterygomaxillary or temporal fossae, base of skull

N - Regional Lymph Nodes

See definitions p. 14.

M - Distant Metastasis

See definitions p. 14.

pTNM Pathological Classification

The pT, pN and pM categories correspond to the T, N and M categories.

G Histopathological Grading

See definitions p. 15.

Stage Grouping

Stage 0	Tis	N0	M0
Stage I	T1	N0	M0
Stage II	T2	N0	M0
Stage III	T3	N0	M0
	T1	N1	M0
	T2	N1	M0
	T3	N1	M0
Stage IV	T4	N0, N1	M0
	Any T	N2, N3	M0
	Any T	Any N	M1

Summary

Maxillary Sinus	
T1	Antral mucosa
T2	Infrastructure, hard palate, nose
T3	Cheek, floor of orbit, ethmoid, posterior wall of sinus
T4	Orbital contents and other adjacent structures
N1	Ipsilateral single $\leqslant 3$ cm
N2	Ipsilateral single > 3 to 6 cm
	Ipsilateral multiple $\leqslant 6$ cm
	Bilateral, contralateral $\leqslant 6$ cm
N3	> 6 cm

Salivary Glands (ICD-O 142)

Rules for Classification

The classification applies only to carcinoma. There should be histological confirmation of the disease.

The following are the procedures for assessment of the T, N and M categories:

T categories   Physical examination and imaging
N categories   Physical examination and imaging
M categories   Physical examination and imaging

Regional Lymph Nodes

The regional lymph nodes are the cervical nodes.

TNM Clinical Classification

T – Primary Tumour

TX   Primary tumour cannot be assessed
T0   No evidence of primary tumour

T1   Tumour 2 cm or less in greatest dimension
T2   Tumour more than 2 cm but not more than 4 cm in greatest dimension
T3   Tumour more than 4 cm but not more than 6 cm in greatest dimension
T4   Tumour more than 6 cm in greatest dimension

Note: All categories are subdivided: (a) no local extension, (b) local extension. Local extension is clinical or macroscopic evidence of invasion of skin, soft tissues, bone, or nerve. Microscopic evidence alone is not local extension for classification purposes.

N – Regional Lymph Nodes

See definitions p. 14.

M – Distant Metastasis

See definitions p. 14.

pTNM Pathological Classification

The pT, pN and pM categories correspond to the T, N and M categories.

G Histopathological Grading

See definitions p. 15.

Stage Grouping

Stage I	T1a	N0	M0
	T2a	N0	M0
Stage II	T1b	N0	M0
	T2b	N0	M0
	T3a	N0	M0
Stage III	T3b	N0	M0
	T4a	N0	M0
	Any T (except T4b)	N1	M0
Stage IV	T4b	Any N	M0
	Any T	N2, N3	M0
	Any T	Any N	M1

Summary

Salivary Glands		
T1	≤ 2 cm	Categories divided:
T2	> 2 to 4 cm	(a) no extension
T3	> 4 to 6 cm	(b) extension
T4	> 6 cm	
N1	Ipsilateral single ≤ 3 cm	
N2	Ipsilateral single > 3 to 6 cm	
	Ipsilateral multiple ≤ 6 cm	
	Bilateral, contralateral ≤ 6 cm	
N3	> 6 cm	

Thyroid Gland (ICD-O 193)

Rules for classification

The classification applies only to carcinoma. There should be histological confirmation of the disease to permit division of cases by histological type.

The following are the procedures for assessment of the T, N and M categories:

T categories	Physical examination, endoscopy and imaging
N categories	Physical examination and imaging
M categories	Physical examination and imaging

Regional Lymph Nodes

The regional lymph nodes are the cervical and upper mediastinal nodes.

TNM Clinical Classification

T – Primary Tumour

TX   Primary tumour cannot be assessed
T0   No evidence of primary tumour

T1   Tumour 1 cm or less in greatest dimension, limited to the thyroid
T2   Tumour more than 1 cm but not more than 4 cm in greatest dimension, limited to the thyroid

T3   Tumour more than 4 cm in greatest dimension, limited to
      the thyroid
T4   Tumour of any size extending beyond the thyroid capsule

Note: All categories may be subdivided: (a) solitary tumour, (b) multifocal
tumour (the largest determines the classification)

N – Regional Lymph Nodes

NX   Regional lymph nodes cannot be assessed
N0   No regional lymph node metastasis
N1   Regional lymph node metastasis
      N1a   Metastasis in ipsilateral cervical lymph node(s)
      N1b   Metastasis in bilateral, midline or contralateral cer-
             vical or mediastinal lymph node(s)

M – Distant Metastasis

See definitions p. 14.

pTNM Pathological Classification

The pT, pN and pM categories correspond to the T, N and M
categories.

Stage Grouping

Papillary or Follicular

	under 45 years			45 years and over		
Stage I	Any T	Any N	M0	T1	N0	M0
Stage II	Any T	Any N	M1	T2	N0	M0
				T3	N0	M0
Stage III	–			T4	N0	M0
				Any T	N1	M0
Stage IV	–			Any T	Any N	M1

Medullary

Stage I	T1	N0	M0
Stage II	T2	N0	M0
	T3	N0	M0
	T4	N0	M0
Stage III	Any T	N1	M0
Stage IV	Any T	Any N	M1

Undifferentiated

Stage IV	Any T Any N Any M
	(all cases are stage IV)

Summary

Thyroid Gland	
T1	$\leqslant 1$ cm
T2	> 1 to 4 cm
T3	> 4 cm
T4	Extends beyond gland
N1	Regional

DIGESTIVE SYSTEM TUMOURS

Introductory Notes

The following sites are included:

Oesophagus	Gall bladder
Stomach	Extrahepatic bile ducts
Colon and rectum	Ampulla of vater
Anal canal	Pancreas (excluding endocrine)
Liver	

Each site is described under the following headings:
Rules for classification with the procedures for assessing the T, N and M categories. Additional methods may be used when they enhance the accuracy of appraisal before treatment
Anatomical sites and subsites where appropriate
Definition of the regional lymph nodes
TNM Clinical classification
pTNM Pathological classification
G Histopathological grading
Stage grouping
Summary

Additional Descriptors

When appropriate, the y symbol, the r symbol and the C-factor category may be added (see p.9).

Distant Metastasis

The definitions of the M categories for all digestive system tumours are:

M – Distant Metastasis

MX   Presence of distant metastasis cannot be assessed
M0   No distant metastasis
M1   Distant metastasis
   The categories M1 and pM1 may be further specified according to the following notation:

Pulmonary	PUL	Bone marrow	MAR
Osseous	OSS	Pleura	PLE
Hepatic	HEP	Peritoneum	PER
Brain	BRA	Skin	SKI
Lymph nodes	LYM	Others	OTH

Histopathological Grading

The definitions of the G categories apply to all digestive system tumours. These are:

G – Histopathological Grading

GX   Grade of differentiation cannot be assessed
G1   Well differentiated
G2   Moderately differentiated
G3   Poorly differentiated
G4   Undifferentiated

R Classification

The absence or presence of residual tumour after treatment may be described by the symbol R. The definitions of the R classification apply to all digestive system tumours. These are:

RX   Presence of residual tumour cannot be assessed
R0   No residual tumour
R1   Microscopic residual tumour
R2   Macroscopic residual tumour

Oesophagus (ICD-O 150)

Rules for classification

The classification applies only to carcinoma. There should be histological confirmation of the disease.

The following are the procedures for assessment of the T, N and M categories:

T categories	Physical examination, imaging, endoscopy (including bronchoscopy) and/or surgical exploration
N categories	Physical examination, imaging and/or surgical exploration
M categories	Physical examination, imaging and/or surgical exploration

Anatomical Subsites

1. Cervical oesophagus (150.0): This commences at the lower border of the cricoid cartilage and ends at the thoracic inlet (suprasternal notch), approximately 18 cm from the upper incisor teeth
2. Intrathoracic oesophagus
   i)   The upper thoracic portion (150.3) extending from the thoracic inlet to the level of the tracheal bifurcation, approximately 24 cm from the upper incisor teeth
   ii) The mid-thoracic portion (150.4) is the proximal half of the oesophagus between the tracheal bifurcation and the oesophagogastric junction. The lower level is approximately 32 cm from the upper incisor teeth
   iii) The lower thoracic portion (150.5), approximately 8 cm in length (includes abdominal oesophagus), is the distal half

of the oesophagus between the tracheal bifurcation and the oesophagogastric junction. The lower level is approximately 40 cm from the upper incisor teeth

Regional Lymph Nodes

The regional lymph nodes are, for the cervical oesophagus, the cervical nodes including supraclavicular nodes, and for the intrathoracic oesophagus, the mediastinal and perigastric nodes, excluding the coeliac nodes.

TNM Clinical Classification

T – Primary Tumour

TX   Primary tumour cannot be assessed
T0   No evidence of primary tumour
Tis   Carcinoma in situ

T1   Tumour invades lamina propria or submucosa
T2   Tumour invades muscularis propria
T3   Tumour invades adventitia
T4   Tumour invades adjacent structures

N – Regional Lymph Nodes

NX   Regional lymph nodes cannot be assessed
N0   No regional lymph node metastasis
N1   Regional lymph node metastasis

M – Distant Metastasis

See definitions p.38.

pTNM Pathological Classification

The pT, pN and pM categories correspond to the T, N and M categories.

G Histopathological Grading

See definitions p. 38.

Stage Grouping

Stage 0	Tis	N0	M0
Stage I	T1	N0	M0
Stage IIA	T2	N0	M0
	T3	N0	M0
Stage IIB	T1	N1	M0
	T2	N1	M0
Stage III	T3	N1	M0
	T4	Any N	M0
Stage IV	Any T	Any N	M1

Summary

Oesophagus	
T1	Lamina propria, submucosa
T2	Muscularis propria
T3	Adventitia
T4	Adjacent structures
N1	Regional

Stomach (ICD-O 151)

Rules for Classification

The classification applies only to carcinoma. There should be histological confirmation of the disease.

The following are the procedures for assessment of T, N and M categories:

T categories Physical examination, imaging, endoscopy, biopsy and/or surgical exploration

N categories Physical examination, imaging and/or surgical exploration

M categories Physical examination, imaging and/or surgical exploration

Anatomical Subsites

1. Upper third: includes the cardiac area (151.0) and fundus (151.3)
2. Middle third: includes the bulk of the corpus (151.4)
3. Lower third: includes the pylorus (151.1) and antral area (151.2)

To delimit these subsites the lesser and greater curvatures are divided at two equidistant points and these are joined. The tumour is assigned to the region in which the bulk of it is situated.

Regional Lymph Nodes

The regional lymph nodes are the perigastric nodes along the lesser and greater curvatures and the nodes located along the left gastric, common hepatic, splenic and coeliac arteries. Involvement of other intra-abdominal lymph nodes such as the hepato-duodenal, retropancreatic, mesenteric and para-aortic is classified as distant metastasis.

TNM Clinical Classification

T – Primary Tumour

TX   Primary tumour cannot be assessed
T0   No evidence of primary tumour
Tis   Carcinoma in situ: intraepithelial tumour without invasion of the lamina propria

T1   Tumour invades lamina propria or submucosa
T2   Tumour invades muscularis propria or subserosa[1]
T3   Tumour penetrates the serosa (visceral peritoneum) without invasion of adjacent structures[2,3]
T4   Tumour invades adjacent structures[2,3]

Notes: 1. A tumour may penetrate muscularis propria with extension into the gastrocolic or gastrohepatic ligaments or the greater or lesser omentum without perforation of the visceral peritoneum covering these structures. In this case, the tumour is classified T2. If there is perforation of the visceral peritoneum covering the gastric ligaments or omenta, the tumour is classified T3.
2. The adjacent structures of the stomach are the spleen, transverse colon, liver, diaphragm, pancreas, abdominal wall, adrenal gland, kidney, small intestine and retroperitoneum.
3. Intramural extension to the duodenum or oesophagus is classified by the depth of greatest invasion in any of these sites including stomach

N – Regional Lymph Nodes

NX   Regional lymph nodes cannot be assessed
N0   No regional lymph node metastasis
N1   Metastasis in perigastric lymph node(s) within 3 cm of the edge of the primary tumour
N2   Metastasis in perigastric lymph node(s) more than 3 cm

from the edge of the primary tumour or in lymph nodes
along the left gastric, common hepatic, splenic or coeliac
arteries

M – Distant Metastasis

See definitions p.38.

pTNM Pathological Classification

The pT, pN and pM categories correspond to the T, N and M
categories.

G Histopathological Grading

See definitions p.38.

Stage Grouping

Stage 0	Tis	N0	M0
Stage IA	T1	N0	M0
Stage IB	T1	N1	M0
	T2	N0	M0
Stage II	T1	N2	M0
	T2	N1	M0
	T3	N0	M0
Stage IIIA	T2	N2	M0
	T3	N1	M0
	T4	N0	M0
Stage IIIB	T3	N2	M0
	T4	N1	M0
Stage IV	T4	N2	M0
	Any T	Any N	M1

Summary

Stomach	
T1	Lamina propria, submucosa
T2	Muscularis propria, subserosa
T3	Penetrates serosa
T4	Adjacent structures
N1	Perigastric ≤ 3 cm from primary
N2	> 3 cm from primary, along left gastric, common hepatic, splenic or coeliac arteries

Colon and Rectum (ICD-O 153, 154.0,1)

Rules for Classification

The classification applies only to carcinoma. There should be histological confirmation of the disease.

The following are the procedures for assessment of the T, N and M categories:

T categories   Physical examination, imaging, endoscopy and/or surgical exploration

N categories   Physical examination, imaging and/or surgical exploration

M categories   Physical examination, imaging and/or surgical exploration

Anatomical Sites and Subsites

Colon

1. Appendix (153.5)
2. Caecum (153.4)
3. Ascending colon (153.6)
4. Hepatic flexure (153.0)
5. Transverse colon (153.1)
6. Splenic flexure (153.7)
7. Descending colon (153.2)
8. Sigmoid colon (153.3)

Rectum

1. Rectosigmoid junction (154.0)
2. Rectum (154.1)

Regional Lymph Nodes

The regional lymph nodes are the pericolic and perirectal and those located along the ileocolic, right colic, middle colic, left colic, inferior mesenteric and superior rectal (haemorrhoidal) arteries.

TNM Clinical Classification

T – Primary Tumour

TX   Primary tumour cannot be assessed
T0   No evidence of primary tumour
Tis   Carcinoma in situ

T1   Tumour invades submucosa
T2   Tumour invades muscularis propria
T3   Tumour invades through muscularis propria into subserosa or into non-peritonealized pericolic or perirectal tissues
T4   Tumour perforates the visceral peritoneum or directly invades other organs or structures

Note: Direct invasion in T4 includes invasion of other segments of the colorectum by way of the serosa, e.g. invasion of the sigmoid colon by a carcinoma of the caecum.

N – Regional Lymph Nodes

NX   Regional lymph nodes cannot be assessed
N0   No regional lymph node metastasis
N1   Metastasis in 1 to 3 pericolic or perirectal lymph nodes
N2   Metastasis in 4 or more pericolic or perirectal lymph nodes
N3   Metastasis in any lymph node along the course of a named vascular trunk

M – Distant Metastasis

See definitions p. 38.

pTNM Pathological Classification

The pT, pN and pM categories correspond to the T, N and M categories.

G Histopathological Grading

See definitions p. 38.

Stage Grouping

				Dukes
Stage 0	Tis	N0	M0	
Stage I	T1	N0	M0	} A
	T2	N0	M0	
Stage II	T3	N0	M0	} B[1]
	T4	N0	M0	
Stage III	Any T	N1	M0	} C[1]
	Any T	N2, N3	M0	
Stage IV	Any T	Any N	M1	

Note: 1. Dukes B is a composite of better (T3N0M0) and worse (T4N0M0) prognostic groups, as is Dukes C (anyTN1M0 and anyTN2,3M0).

Summary

Colon, Rectum	
T1	Submucosa
T2	Muscularis propria
T3	Subserosa, non-peritonealized pericolic/perirectal tissues
T4	Visceral peritoneum/other organs or structures
N1	≤ 3 pericolic/perirectal
N2	> 3 pericolic/perirectal
N3	Nodes on named vascular trunk

Anal Canal (ICD-O 154.2)

The anal canal extends from the rectum to the perianal skin (to the junction with hair-bearing skin). It is lined by the mucous membrane overlying the internal sphincter, including the transitional epithelium and dentate line. Tumours of the anal margin (ICD-O 173.5) are classified with skin tumours (p. 83).

Rules for Classification

The classification applies only to carcinoma. There should be histological confirmation of the disease.

The following are the procedures for assessment of T, N and M categories:

T categories   Physical examination, imaging and endoscopy
N categories   Physical examination and imaging
M categories   Physical examination and imaging

Regional Lymph Nodes

The regional lymph nodes are the perirectal, internal iliac and the inguinal lymph nodes.

TNM Clinical Classification

T – Primary Tumour

TX   Primary tumour cannot be assessed
T0   No evidence of primary tumour
Tis   Carcinoma in situ

T1   Tumour 2 cm or less in greatest dimension
T2   Tumour more than 2 cm but not more than 5 cm in greatest
      dimension
T3   Tumour more than 5 cm in greatest dimension
T4   Tumour of any size invades adjacent organ(s), e.g. vagina,
      urethra, bladder (involvement of the sphincter muscle(s)
      alone is not classified T4)

N - Regional Lymph Nodes

NX   Regional lymph nodes cannot be assessed
N0   No regional lymph node metastasis
N1   Metastasis in perirectal lymph node(s)
N2   Metastasis in unilateral internal iliac and/or inguinal
      lymph node(s)
N3   Metastasis in perirectal and inguinal lymph nodes and/or
      bilateral internal iliac and/or inguinal lymph nodes

M - Distant Metastasis

See definitions p. 38.

pTNM Pathological Classification

The pT, pN and pM categories correspond to the T, N and M
categories.

G Histopathological Grading

See definitions p. 38.

Stage Grouping

Stage 0	Tis	N0	M0
Stage I	T1	N0	M0
Stage II	T2	N0	M0
	T3	N0	M0
Stage IIIA	T4	N0	M0
	T1	N1	M0
	T2	N1	M0
	T3	N1	M0
Stage IIIB	T4	N1	M0
	Any T	N2, N3	M0
Stage IV	Any T	Any N	M1

Summary

Anal Canal	
T1	≤ 2 cm
T2	> 2 to 5 cm
T3	> 5 cm
T4	Adjacent organ(s)
N1	Perirectal
N2	Unilateral internal iliac/inguinal
N3	Perirectal and inguinal, bilateral internal iliac/inguinal

Liver (ICD-O 155)

Rules for Classification

The classification applies only to primary hepatocellular and cholangio- (intrahepatic bile duct) carcinoma of the liver. There should be histological confirmation of the disease.

The following are the procedures for assessment of the T, N and M categories:

T categories	Physical examination, imaging and/or surgical exploration
N categories	Physical examination, imaging and/or surgical exploration
M categories	Physical examination, imaging and/or surgical exploration

Note: Although the presence of cirrhosis is an important prognostic factor it does not affect the TNM classification, being an independent variable.

Anatomical Subsites

1. Liver (155.0)
2. Intrahepatic bile duct (155.1)

Regional Lymph Nodes

The regional lymph nodes are the hilar nodes (i.e. in the hepato-duodenal ligament).

TNM Clinical Classification

T – Primary Tumour

TX   Primary tumour cannot be assessed
T0   No evidence of primary tumour

T1   Solitary tumour 2 cm or less in greatest dimension without
      vascular invasion
T2   Solitary tumour 2 cm or less in greatest dimension with
      vascular invasion, *or* multiple tumours limited to one lobe
      none more than 2 cm in greatest dimension without vascu-
      lar invasion, *or* solitary tumour more than 2 cm in greatest
      dimension without vascular invasion
T3   Solitary tumour more than 2 cm in greatest dimension with
      vascular invasion, *or* multiple tumours limited to one lobe
      none more than 2 cm in greatest dimension with vascular
      invasion, *or* multiple tumours limited to one lobe, any
      more than 2 cm in greatest dimension with or without vas-
      cular invasion
T4   Multiple tumours in more than one lobe, *or* tumour(s)
      involve(s) a major branch of the portal or hepatic vein(s)

Note: For classification, the plane projecting between the bed of the gall
bladder and the inferior vena cava divides the liver in two lobes.

N – Regional Lymph Nodes

NX   Regional lymph nodes cannot be assessed
N0   No regional lymph node metastasis
N1   Regional lymph node metastasis

M – Distant Metastasis

See definitions p. 38.

pTNM Pathological Classification

The pT, pN and pM categories correspond to the T, N and M categories.

G Histopathological Grading

See definitions p. 38.

Stage Grouping

Stage I	T1	N0	M0
Stage II	T2	N0	M0
Stage III	T1	N1	M0
	T2	N1	M0
	T3	N0, N1	M0
Stage IVA	T4	Any N	M0
Stage IVB	Any T	Any N	M1

Summary

Liver	
T1	Solitary, ≤ 2 cm, without vascular invasion
T2	Solitary, ≤ 2 cm, with vascular invasion
	Multiple, one lobe, ≤ 2 cm, without vascular invasion
	Solitary, > 2 cm, without vascular invasion
T3	Solitary, > 2 cm, with vascular invasion
	Multiple, one lobe, ≤ 2 cm, with vascular invasion
	Multiple, one lobe, > 2 cm, with or without vascular invasion
T4	Multiple, > one lobe
	Invasion of major branch of portal or hepatic veins
N1	Regional

Gall Bladder (ICD-O 156.0)

Rules for Classification

The classification applies only to carcinoma. There should be histological confirmation of the disease.

The following are the procedures for assessment of the T, N and M categories:

T categories Physical examination, imaging and/or surgical exploration

N categories Physical examination, imaging and/or surgical exploration

M categories Physical examination, imaging and/or surgical exploration

Regional Lymph Nodes

The regional lymph nodes are the cystic duct node and the pericholedochal, hilar, peripancreatic (head only), periduodenal, periportal, coeliac and superior mesenteric nodes.

TNM Clinical Classification

T – Primary Tumour

TX   Primary tumour cannot be assessed
T0   No evidence of primary tumour
Tis   Carcinoma in situ

T1   Tumour invades mucosa or muscle layer
    T1a   Tumour invades mucosa
    T1b   Tumour invades muscle layer

T2   Tumour invades perimuscular connective tissue, no exten-
      sion beyond serosa or into liver
T3   Tumour invades beyond serosa or into one adjacent organ
      or both (extension 2 cm or less into liver)
T4   Tumour extends more than 2 cm into liver and/or into two
      or more adjacent organs (stomach, duodenum, colon, pan-
      creas, omentum, extrahepatic bile ducts, any involvement
      of liver)

N – Regional Lymph Nodes

NX   Regional lymph nodes cannot be assessed
N0   No regional lymph node metastasis
N1   Regional lymph node metastasis
      N1a   Metastasis in cystic duct, pericholedochal, and/or
             hilar lymph nodes (i. e. in the hepatoduodenal liga-
             ment)
      N1b   Metastasis in peripancreatic (head only), periduo-
             denal, periportal, coeliac and/or superior mesen-
             teric lymph nodes

M – Distant Metastasis

See definitions p. 38.

pTNM Pathological Classification

The pT, pN and pM categories correspond to the T, N and
M categories.

G Histopathological Grading

See definitions p. 38.

Stage Grouping

Stage 0	Tis	N0	M0
Stage I	T1	N0	M0
Stage II	T2	N0	M0
Stage III	T1	N1	M0
	T2	N1	M0
	T3	Any N	M0
Stage IV	T4	Any N	M0
	Any T	Any N	M1

Summary

Gall Bladder	
T1	Gall bladder wall
T1a	Mucosa
T1b	Muscle
T2	Perimuscular connective tissue
T3	Serosa and/or one organ, liver ≤ 2 cm
T4	Two or more organs, or liver > 2 cm
N1a	Hepatoduodenal ligament
N1b	Other regional

Extrahepatic Bile Ducts (ICD-O 156.1)

Rules for Classification

The classification applies only to carcinoma. There should be histological confirmation of the disease.

The following are the procedures for assessment of the T, N and M categories:

T categories Physical examination, imaging and/or surgical exploration
N categories Physical examination, imaging and/or surgical exploration
M categories Physical examination, imaging and/or surgical exploration

Regional Lymph Nodes

The regional lymph nodes are the cystic duct, pericholedochal, hilar, peripancreatic (head only), periduodenal, periportal, coeliac and superior mesenteric nodes.

TNM Clinical Classification

T – Primary Tumour

TX   Primary tumour cannot be assessed
T0   No evidence of primary tumour
Tis   Carcinoma in situ

T1   Tumour invades mucosa or muscle layer
      T1a   Tumour invades mucosa
      T1b   Tumour invades muscle layer
T2   Tumour invades perimuscular connective tissue

T3   Tumour invades adjacent structures: liver, pancreas, duo-
        denum, gallbladder, colon, stomach

N – Regional Lymph Nodes

NX   Regional lymph nodes cannot be assessed
N0   No regional lymph node metastasis
N1   Regional lymph node metastasis
        N1a   Metastasis in cystic duct, pericholedochal and/or
                hilar lymph nodes (i.e. in the hepatoduodenal liga-
                ment)
        N1b   Metastasis in peripancreatic (head only), periduo-
                denal, periportal, coeliac and/or superior mesen-
                teric lymph nodes

M – Distant Metastasis

See definitions p. 38.

pTNM Pathological Classification

The pT, pN and pM categories correspond to the T, N and M
categories.

G Histopathological Grading

See definitions p. 38.

Stage Grouping

Stage 0	Tis	N0	M0
Stage I	T1	N0	M0
Stage II	T2	N0	M0
Stage III	T1	N1	M0
	T2	N1	M0
Stage IVA	T3	Any N	M0
Stage IVB	Any T	Any N	M1

Summary

Extrahepatic Bile Ducts	
T1	Ductal wall
T1a	Mucosa
T1b	Muscle
T2	Perimuscular connective tissue
T3	Adjacent structures
N1a	Hepatoduodenal ligament
N1b	Other regional

Ampulla of Vater (ICD-O 156.2)

Rules for Classification

The classification applies only to carcinoma. There should be histological confirmation of the disease.

The following are the procedures for assessment of the T, N and M categories:

T categories	Physical examination, imaging and/or surgical exploration
N categories	Physical examination, imaging and/or surgical exploration
M categories	Physical examination, imaging and/or surgical exploration

Regional Lymph Nodes

The regional lymph nodes are:

Superior	Superior to head and body of the pancreas
Inferior	Inferior to head and body of the pancreas
Anterior	Anterior pancreaticoduodenal, pyloric, and proximal mesenteric lymph nodes
Posterior	Posterior pancreaticoduodenal, common bile duct, and proximal mesenteric

Note: The splenic lymph nodes and those at the tail of the pancreas are *not* regional; metastases to these lymph nodes are coded M1.

TNM Clinical Classification

T – Primary Tumour

TX	Primary tumour cannot be assessed
T0	No evidence of primary tumour
Tis	Carcinoma in situ

T1   Tumour limited to ampulla of Vater
T2   Tumour invades duodenal wall
T3   Tumor invades 2 cm or less into pancreas
T4   Tumour invades more than 2 cm into pancreas and/or into
       other adjacent organs

N – Regional Lymph Nodes

NX   Regional lymph nodes cannot be assessed
N0   No regional lymph node metastasis
N1   Regional lymph node metastasis

M – Distant Metastasis

See definitions p. 38.

pTNM Pathological Classification

The pT, pN and pM categories correspond to the T, N and M
categories.

G Histopathological Grading

See definitions p. 38.

Stage Grouping

Stage 0	Tis	N0	M0
Stage I	T1	N0	M0
Stage II	T2	N0	M0
	T3	N0	M0
Stage III	T1	N1	M0
	T2	N1	M0
	T3	N1	M0
Stage IV	T4	Any N	M0
	Any T	Any N	M1

Summary

Ampulla of Vater	
T1	Ampulla only
T2	Duodenal wall
T3	Pancreas ≤ 2 cm
T4	Pancreas > 2 cm, other organs
N1	Regional

Pancreas (ICD-O 157.0–3)

Rules for Classification

The classification applies only to carcinoma of the exocrine pancreas. There should be histological or cytological confirmation of the disease.

The following are the procedures for assessment of the T, N and M categories:

T categories	Physical examination, imaging and/or surgical exploration
N categories	Physical examination, imaging and/or surgical exploration
M categories	Physical examination, imaging and/or surgical exploration

Anatomical Subsites

1. Head of pancreas[1] (157.0)
2. Body of pancreas[2] (157.1)
3. Tail of pancreas[3] (157.2)
4. Entire pancreas (157.8)

Notes: 1. Tumours of the head of the pancreas are those arising to the right of the left border of the superior mesenteric vein. The uncinate process is considered as part of the head.

2. Tumours of the body are those arising between the left border of the superior mesenteric vein and left border of the aorta.

3. Tumours of the tail are those arising between the left border of the aorta and the hilum of the spleen.

Regional Lymph Nodes

The regional lymph nodes are the peripancreatic nodes which may be subdivided as follows:

Superior	Superior to head and body
Inferior	Inferior to head and body
Anterior	Anterior pancreaticoduodenal, pyloric and proximal mesenteric
Posterior	Posterior pancreaticoduodenal, common bile duct and proximal mesenteric
Splenic	Hilum of spleen and tail of pancreas

TNM Clinical Classification

T - Primary Tumour

TX   Primary tumour cannot be assessed
T0   No evidence of primary tumour

T1   Tumour limited to the pancreas
    T1a   Tumour 2 cm or less in greatest dimension
    T1b   Tumour more than 2 cm in greatest dimension
T2   Tumour extends directly to any of the following: duodenum, bile duct, peripancreatic tissues
T3   Tumour extends directly to any of the following: stomach, spleen, colon, adjacent large vessels

N - Regional Lymph Nodes

NX   Regional lymph nodes cannot be assessed
N0   No regional lymph node metastasis
N1   Regional lymph node metastasis

M - Distant Metastasis

See definitions p. 38.

pTNM Pathological Classification

The pT, pN and pM categories correspond to the T, N and M categories.

G Histopathological Grading

See definitions p.38.

Stage Grouping

Stage I	T1	N0	M0
	T2	N0	M0
Stage II	T3	N0	M0
Stage III	Any T	N1	M0
Stage IV	Any T	Any N	M1

Summary

Pancreas		
T1		Limited to pancreas
	T1a	≤ 2 cm
	T1b	> 2 cm
T2		Duodenum, bile duct, peripancreatic tissues
T3		Stomach, spleen, colon, large vessels
N1		Regional

LUNG TUMOURS (ICD-O 162)

Introductory Notes

The region is described under the following headings:
Rules for classification with the procedures for assessing the T, N and M categories. Additional methods may be used when they enhance the accuracy of appraisal before treatment
Anatomical subsites
Definition of the regional lymph nodes
TNM Clinical classification
pTNM Pathological classification
G Histopathological grading
R classification
Stage grouping
Summary

Rules for Classification

The classification applies only to carcinoma. There should be histological confirmation of the disease to permit division of cases by histological type.

The following are the procedures for assessment of the T, N and M categories:

T categories	Physical examination, imaging, endoscopy and/or surgical exploration
N categories	Physical examination, imaging, endoscopy and/or surgical exploration
M categories	Physical examination, imaging and/or surgical exploration

Additional Descriptors

When appropriate the y symbol, the r symbol and the C-factor category may be added (see p. 9).

Anatomical Subsites

1. Main bronchus (162.2)
2. Upper lobe (162.3)
3. Middle lobe (162.4)
4. Lower lobe (162.5)

Regional Lymph Nodes

The regional lymph nodes are the intrathoracic, scalene and supraclavicular nodes.

TNM Clinical Classification

T – Primary Tumour

TX   Primary tumour cannot be assessed, *or* tumour proven by the pres-
      ence of malignant cells in sputum or bronchial washings but not visu-
      alized by imaging or bronchoscopy
T0   No evidence of primary tumour
Tis   Carcinoma in situ

T1   Tumour 3 cm or less in greatest dimension, surrounded by lung or visceral pleura, without bronchoscopic evidence of invasion more proximal than the lobar bronchus (i.e. not in the main bronchus)[1]
T2   Tumour with *any* of the following features of size or extent:
      More than 3 cm in greatest dimension
      Involves main bronchus, 2 cm or more distal to the carina
      Invades visceral pleura

Associated with atelectasis or obstructive pneumonitis which extends to the hilar region but does not involve the entire lung

T3 Tumour of any size which directly invades any of the following: chest wall (including superior sulcus tumours), diaphragm, mediastinal pleura, parietal pericardium; or tumour in the main bronchus less than 2 cm distal to the carina[1]) but without involvement of the carina; or associated atelectasis or obstructive pneumonitis of the entire lung

T4 Tumour of any size which invades any of the following: mediastinum, heart, great vessels, trachea, oesophagus, vertebral body, carina; or tumour with malignant pleural effusion[2]

Notes: 1. The uncommon superficial spreading tumour of any size with its invasive component limited to the bronchial wall which may extend proximal to the main bronchus is also classified T1.

2. Most pleural effusions associated with lung cancer are due to tumour. However, there are a few patients in whom multiple cytopathological examinations of pleural fluid are negative for tumour, the fluid is non-bloody and is not an exudate. Where these elements and clinical judgment dictate that the effusion is not related to the tumour, the effusion should be excluded as a staging element and the patient should be classified T1, T2 or T3.

N – Regional Lymph Nodes

NX Regional lymph nodes cannot be assessed
N0 No regional lymph node metastasis
N1 Metastasis in ipsilateral peribronchial and/or ipsilateral hilar lymph nodes, including direct extension
N2 Metastasis in ipsilateral mediastinal and/or subcarinal lymph node(s)
N3 Metastasis in contralateral mediastinal, contralateral hilar, ipsilateral or contralateral scalene or supraclavicular lymph node(s)

M – Distant Metastasis

MX   Presence of distant metastasis cannot be assessed
M0   No distant metastasis
M1   Distant metastasis
   The category M1 may be further specified according to the following notation:

Pulmonary	PUL	Bone marrow	MAR
Osseous	OSS	Pleura	PLE
Hepatic	HEP	Peritoneum	PER
Brain	BRA	Skin	SKI
Lymph nodes	LYM	Other	OTH

pTNM Pathological Classification

The pT, pN and pM categories correspond to the T, N and M categories.

G Histopathological Grading

GX   Grade of differentiation cannot be assessed
G1   Well differentiated
G2   Moderately differentiated
G3   Poorly differentiated
G4   Undifferentiated

R Classification

The absence or presence of residual tumour after treatment may be described by the symbol R:
RX   Presence of residual tumour cannot be assessed
R0   No residual tumour
R1   Microscopic residual tumour
R2   Macroscopic residual tumour

Stage Grouping

Occult carcinoma	TX	N0	M0
Stage 0	Tis	N0	M0
Stage I	T1	N0	M0
	T2	N0	M0
Stage II	T1	N1	M0
	T2	N1	M0
Stage IIIA	T1	N2	M0
	T2	N2	M0
	T3	N0, N1, N2	M0
Stage IIIB	Any T	N3	M0
	T4	Any N	M0
Stage IV	Any T	Any N	M1

Summary

Lung	
TX	Positive cytology
T1	≤ 3 cm
T2	> 3 cm/extends to hilar region/invades visceral pleura/partial atelectasis
T3	Chest wall, diaphragm, pericardium, mediastinal pleura etc., total atelectasis
T4	Mediastinum, heart, great vessels, trachea, oesophagus etc., malignant effusion
N1	Peribronchial, ipsilateral hilar
N2	Ipsilateral mediastinal
N3	Contralateral mediastinal, scalene or supraclavicular

TUMOURS OF BONE AND SOFT TISSUES

Introductory Notes

The following sites are included:
Soft tissue
Bone

Each site is described under the following headings:
Rules for classification with the procedures for assessing the T, N and M categories. Additional methods may be used when they enhance the accuracy of appraisal before treatment
Anatomical sites where appropriate
Definition of the regional lymph nodes
TNM Clinical classification
pTNM Pathological classification
G Histopathological grading
Stage grouping
Summary

Additional Descriptors

When appropriate, the y symbol, the r symbol and the C-factor category may be added (see p.9).

Regional Lymph Nodes

The definitions of the N categories for all tumours of bone and soft tissues are:

N – Regional Lymph Nodes

NX   Regional lymph nodes cannot be assessed
N0   No regional lymph node metastasis
N1   Regional lymph node metastasis

Distant Metastasis

The definitions of the M categories for all tumours of bones and soft tissues are:

M – Distant Metastasis

MX   Presence of distant metastasis cannot be assessed
M0   No distant metastasis
M1   Distant metastasis
    The categories M1 and pM1 may be further specified according to the following notation:

Pulmonary	PUL	Bone marrow	MAR
Osseous	OSS	Pleura	PLE
Hepatic	HEP	Peritoneum	PER
Brain	BRA	Skin	SKI
Lymph nodes	LYM	Others	OTH

R Classification

The absence or presence of residual tumour after treatment may be described by the symbol R. The definitions of the R classification apply to all tumours of bones and soft tissues. These are:
RX   Presence of residual tumour cannot be assessed
R0   No residual tumour
R1   Microscopic residual tumour
R2   Macroscopic residual tumour

Bone (ICD-O 170)

Rules for Classification

The classification applies to all primary malignant bone tumours except multiple myeloma, juxtacortical osteosarcoma and juxta-cortical chondrosarcoma. There should be histological confirmation of the disease to permit division of cases by histological type.

The following are the procedures for assessing the T, N and M categories:

T categories   Physical examination and imaging
N categories   Physical examination and imaging
M categories   Physical examination and imaging

Regional Lymph Nodes

The regional lymph nodes are those appropriate to the situation of the primary tumour.

TNM Clinical Classification

T – Primary Tumour

TX   Primary tumour cannot be assessed
T0   No evidence of primary tumour

T1   Tumour confined within the cortex
T2   Tumour invades beyond the cortex

N – Regional Lymph Nodes

See definitions p. 76.

M – Distant Metastasis

See definitions p. 76.

pTNM Pathological Classification

The pT, pN and pM categories correspond to the T, N and M
categories.

G Histopathological Grading

GX   Grade of differentiation cannot be assessed
G1   Well differentiated
G2   Moderately differentiated
G3   Poorly differentiated
G4   Undifferentiated

Note: Ewing's sarcoma and primary lymphoma of bone are defined as G4.

Stage Grouping

Stage IA	G1, 2	T1	N0	M0
Stage IB	G1, 2	T2	N0	M0
Stage IIA	G3, 4	T1	N0	M0
Stage IIB	G3, 4	T2	N0	M0
Stage III	Not defined			
Stage IVA	Any G	Any T	N1	M0
Stage IVB	Any G	Any T	Any N	M1

Summary

Bone	
T1	Within cortex
T2	Beyond cortex
N1	Regional
G1	Well differentiated
G2	Moderately differentiated
G3	Poorly differentiated
G4	Undifferentiated

Soft Tissues (ICD-O 158.0, 164.2,3, 171)

Rules for Classification

There should be histological confirmation of the disease to permit division of cases by histological type.

The following are the procedures for assessing the T, N and M categories:

T categories Physical examination and imaging
N categories Physical examination and imaging
M categories Physical examination and imaging

Anatomical Sites

1. Connective, subcutaneous and other soft tissues (171)
2. Retroperitoneum (158.0)
3. Mediastinum (164.2,3)

Histological Types of Tumour

The following histological types of malignant tumour are included, the appropriate ICD-O morphology rubrics being indicated:

Alveolar soft-part sarcoma	9581/3
Angiosarcoma	9120/3
Epitheloid sarcoma	8804/3
Extraskeletal chondrosarcoma	9220/3
Extraskeletal osteosarcoma	9180/3
Fibrosarcoma	8810/3
Leiomyosarcoma	8890/3
Liposarcoma	8850/3
Malignant fibrous histiocytoma	8830/3
Malignant hemangiopericytoma	9150/3

Malignant mesenchymoma	8990/3
Malignant schwannoma	9560/3
Rhabdomyosarcoma	8900/3
Synovial sarcoma	9040/3
Sarcoma NOS (not otherwise specified)	8800/3

The following histological types of tumours are not included: Kaposi's sarcoma, dermatofibrosarcoma (protuberans), fibrosarcoma grade I (desmoid tumour) and sarcomata arising from the dura mater, brain, parenchymatous organs or hollow viscera.

Regional Lymph Nodes

The regional lymph nodes are those appropriate to the situation of the primary tumour.

TNM Clinical Classification

T - Primary Tumour

TX   Primary tumour cannot be assessed
T0   No evidence of primary tumour

T1   Tumour 5 cm or less in greatest dimension
T2   Tumour more than 5 cm in greatest dimension

N - Regional Lymph Nodes

See definitions p. 76.

M - Distant Metastasis

See definitions p. 76.

pTNM Pathological Classification

The pT, pN and pM categories correspond to the T, N and M categories.

G Histopathological Grading

GX   Grade of differentiation cannot be assessed
G1   Well differentiated
G2   Moderately differentiated
G3-4 Poorly differentiated/undifferentiated

Note: After the histological type has been determined, the tumour should be
graded according to the accepted criteria including cellularity, cellular
pleomorphism, mitotic activity and necrosis. The amount of intercellu-
lar substance such as collagen or mucoid material should be considered as a favourable factor in assessing the grade.

Stage Grouping

Stage IA	G1	T1	N0	M0
Stage IB	G1	T2	N0	M0
Stage IIA	G2	T1	N0	M0
Stage IIB	G2	T2	N0	M0
Stage IIIA	G3-4	T1	N0	M0
Stage IIIB	G3-4	T2	N0	M0
Stage IVA	Any G	Any T	N1	M0
Stage IVB	Any G	Any T	Any N	M1

Summary

Soft Tissue Sarcoma	
T1	≤ 5 cm
T2	> 5 cm
N1	Regional
G1	Well differentiated
G2	Moderately differentiated
G3-4	Poorly differentiated/undifferentiated

SKIN TUMOURS

Introductory Notes

The classification applies to carcinoma of the skin excluding eyelid (see p. 148), vulva (see p. 118) and penis (see p. 130), and to melanoma of the skin.

Anatomical Sites

The following sites are identified by ICD-O topography rubrics:
1. Lip (excluding vermilion surface) (173.0)
2. Eyelid (173.1)
3. External ear (173.2)
4. Other parts of face (173.3)
5. Scalp and neck (173.4)
6. Trunk including anal margin and perianal skin (173.5)
7. Arm and shoulder (173.6)
8. Leg and hip (173.7)
9. Scrotum (187.7)

Each tumour type is described under the following headings:
Rules for classification with the procedures for assessing the T, N and M categories
Regional lymph nodes
TNM Clinical classification
pTNM Pathological classification
G Histopathological grading where applicable
Stage grouping
Summary

Additional Descriptors

When appropriate, the y symbol, the r symbol and the C-factor category may be added (see p.9).

Regional Lymph Nodes

The regional lymph nodes are those appropriate to the situation of the primary tumour.

Unilateral Tumours

Head, neck	Ipsilateral preauricular, submandibular, cervical and supraclavicular lymph nodes
Thorax	Ipsilateral axillary lymph nodes
Arm	Ipsilateral epitrochlear and axillary lymph nodes
Abdomen, loins and buttocks	Ipsilateral inguinal lymph nodes
Leg	Ipsilateral popliteal and inguinal lymph nodes
Anal margin and peri-anal skin	Ipsilateral inguinal lymph nodes

Tumours in the Boundary Zones Between the Above

The lymph nodes pertaining to the regions on both sides of the boundary zone are considered to be regional lymph nodes. The following 4-cm-wide bands are considered as boundary zones:

Between	*Along*
Right/left	Midline
Head and neck/thorax	Clavicula-acromion-upper shoulder blade edge
Thorax/arm	Shoulder-axilla-shoulder

Thorax/abdomen, loins and buttocks	*Front:*	middle between navel and costal arch
	Back:	lower border of thoracic vertebrae (midtransverse axis)
Abdomen, loins and buttock/leg		Groin-trochanter-gluteal sulcus

Any metastasis to other than the listed regional lymph nodes is considered M1.

Distant Metastasis

The definitions of the M categories for all skin tumours are:

M – Distant Metastasis

MX   Presence of distant metastasis cannot be assessed
M0   No distant metastasis
M1   Distant metastasis
   The categories M1 and pM1 may be further specified according to the following notation:

Pulmonary	PUL	Bone marrow	MAR
Osseous	OSS	Pleura	PLE
Hepatic	HEP	Peritoneum	PER
Brain	BRA	Skin	SKI
Lymph nodes	LYM	Other	OTH

R Classification

The absence or presence of residual tumour after treatment may be described by the symbol R. The definitions of the R classification apply to all skin tumour types. These are:

RX   Presence of residual tumour cannot be assessed
R0   No residual tumour
R1   Microscopic residual tumour
R2   Macroscopic residual tumour

Carcinoma of Skin (excluding eyelid, vulva and penis) (ICD-O 173, 187.7)

Rules for Classification

The classification applies only to carcinoma. There should be histological confirmation of the disease to permit division of cases by histological type.

The following are the procedures for assessment of the T, N and M categories:

T categories	Physical examination
N categories	Physical examination and imaging
M categories	Physical examination and imaging

Regional Lymph Nodes

See p. 84.

TNM Clinical Classification

T – Primary Tumour

TX   Primary tumour cannot be assessed
T0   No evidence of primary tumour
Tis   Carcinoma in situ

T1   Tumour 2 cm or less in greatest dimension
T2   Tumour more than 2 cm but not more than 5 cm in greatest dimension
T3   Tumour more than 5 cm in greatest dimension
T4   Tumour invades deep extradermal structures, i. e. cartilage, skeletal muscle or bone

Note: In the case of multiple simultaneous tumours, the tumour with the highest T category will be classified and the number of separate tumours will be indicated in parenthesis, e.g. T2 (5).

N – Regional Lymph Nodes

NX   Regional lymph nodes cannot be assessed
N0   No regional lymph node metastasis
N1   Regional lymph node metastasis

M – Distant Metastasis

See definitions p.85.

pTNM Pathological Classification

The pT, pN and pM categories correspond to the T, N and M categories.

G Histopathological Grading

GX   Grade of differentiation cannot be assessed
G1   Well differentiated
G2   Moderately differentiated
G3   Poorly differentiated
G4   Undifferentiated

Stage Grouping

Stage 0	Tis	N0	M0
Stage I	T1	N0	M0
Stage II	T2	N0	M0
	T3	N0	M0
Stage III	T4	N0	M0
	Any T	N1	M0
Stage IV	Any T	Any N	M1

Summary

Skin Carcinoma	
T1	$\leqslant 2$ cm
T2	> 2 to 5 cm
T3	> 5 cm
T4	Deep extradermal structures (cartilage, skeletal muscle, bone)
N1	Regional

Melanoma of Skin
(ICD-O 173, 184.4, 187.4, 187.7)

Rules for Classification

There should be histological confirmation of the disease.
  The following are the procedures for assessment of the N and M categories.

N categories	Physical examination and imaging
M categories	Physical examination and imaging

Regional Lymph Nodes

See p. 84.

TNM Clinical Classification

T – Primary Tumour

The extent of tumour is classified after excision, see pT, p. 90.

N – Regional Lymph Nodes

NX   Regional lymph nodes cannot be assessed
N0   No regional lymph node metastasis
N1   Metastasis 3 cm or less in greatest dimension in any regional lymph node(s)
N2   Metastasis more than 3 cm in greatest dimension in any regional lymph node(s) and/or in-transit metastasis
    N2a   Metastasis more than 3 cm in greatest dimension in any regional node(s)
    N2b   In-transit metastasis
    N2c   Both

Note: In-transit metastasis involves skin or subcutaneous tissue more than 2 cm from the primary tumour not beyond the regional lymph nodes.

M – Distant Metastasis

MX   Presence of distant metastasis cannot be assessed
M0   No distant metastasis
M1   Distant metastasis
    M1a   Metastasis in skin or subcutaneous tissue or lymph
            node(s) beyond the regional lymph nodes
    M1b   Visceral metastasis

pTNM Pathological Classification

pT – Primary Tumour

pTX   Primary tumour cannot be assessed
pT0   No evidence of primary tumour
pTis   Melanoma in situ (Clark's level I) (atypical melanocytic hyperplasia, severe melanocytic dysplasia, not an invasive malignant lesion)

pT1   Tumour 0.75 mm or less in thickness and invades the papillary dermis (Clark's level II)

pT2   Tumour more than 0.75 mm but not more than 1.5 mm in thickness and/or invades to the papillary-reticular dermal interface (Clark's level III)

pT3   Tumour more than 1.5 mm but not more than 4.0 mm in thickness and/or invades the reticular dermis (Clark's level IV)
    pT3a   Tumour more than 1.5 mm but not more than 3.0 mm in thickness
    pT3b   Tumour more than 3.0 mm but not more than 4.0 mm in thickness

pT4   Tumour more than 4.0 mm in thickness and/or invades subcutaneous tissue (Clark's level V) and/or satellite(s) within 2 cm of the primary tumour
    pT4a   Tumour more than 4.0 mm in thickness and/or invades subcutaneous tissue
    pT4b   Satellite(s) within 2 cm of the primary tumour

Note: In case of discrepancy between tumour thickness and level, the pT category is based on the less favourable finding.

pN – Regional Lymph Nodes

The pN categories correspond to the N categories.

pM – Distant Metastasis

The pM categories correspond to the M categories.

Stage Grouping

Stage I	pT1	N0	M0
	pT2	N0	M0
Stage II	pT3	N0	M0
Stage III	pT4	N0	M0
	Any pT	N1, N2	M0
Stage IV	Any pT	Any N	M1

Summary

Skin Melanoma		
pT1	≤ 0.75 mm	Level II
pT2	> 0.75 to 1.5 mm	Level III
pT3	> 1.5 to 4 mm	Level IV
pT4	> 4.0 mm/satellites	Level V
N1	Regional ≤ 3 cm	
N2	Regional > 3 cm and/or in-transit metastasis	

BREAST TUMOURS (ICD-O 174)

Introductory Notes

The site is described under the following headings:

Rules for classification with the procedures for determining the
T, N and M categories. Additional methods may be used when
they enhance the accuracy of appraisal before treatment
Anatomical subsites
Definitions of the regional lymph nodes
TNM Clinical classification
pTNM Pathological classification
G Histopathological grading
R classification
Stage grouping
Summary

Rules for Classification

The classification applies only to carcinoma. There should be
histological confirmation of the disease. The anatomical subsite
of origin should be recorded but is not considered in classification.

In the case of multiple simultaneous tumours in one breast, the
tumour with the highest T category should be used for classification. Simultaneous *bilateral* breast cancers should be classified
independently.

The following are the procedures for assessment of T, N and
M categories:

T categories   Physical examination and imaging, e.g. mammo-
                 graphy

N categories   Physical examination and imaging
M categories   Physical examination and imaging

Additional Descriptors

When appropriate, the y symbol, the r symbol and the C-factor category may be added (see p. 9).

Anatomical Subsites

1. Nipple (174.0)
2. Central portion (174.1)
3. Upper-inner quadrant (174.2)
4. Lower-inner quadrant (174.3)
5. Upper-outer quadrant (174.4)
6. Lower-outer quadrant (174.5)
7. Axillary tail (174.6)

Regional Lymph Nodes

The regional lymph nodes are:
1. *Axillary* (ipsilateral) and *interpectoral* (Rotter's nodes): lymph nodes along the axillary vein and its tributaries, which may be divided into the following levels:
   i)   *Level I* (low-axilla): lymph nodes lateral to the lateral border of pectoralis minor muscle.
   ii) *Level II* (mid-axilla): lymph nodes between the medial and lateral borders of the pectoralis minor muscle and the interpectoral (Rotter's) lymph nodes.
   iii) *Level III* (apical axilla): lymph nodes medial to the medial margin of the pectoralis minor muscle including those designated as the subclavicular, infraclavicular, or apical.

   Note: Intramammary lymph nodes are coded as axillary lymph nodes.

2. *Internal mammary* (ipsilateral): lymph nodes in the intercostal spaces along the edge of the sternum in the endothoracic fascia.

Any other lymph node metastasis is coded as a distant metastasis (M1), including supraclavicular, cervical, or contralateral internal mammary lymph nodes.

TNM Clinical Classification

TX   Primary tumour cannot be assessed
TO   No evidence of primary tumour
Tis Carcinoma in situ: intraductal carcinoma, or lobular carcinoma in situ, or Paget's disease of the nipple with no tumour

Note: Paget's disease associated with a tumour is classified according to the size of the tumour.

T1   Tumour 2 cm or less in greatest dimension
    T1a   0.5 cm or less in greatest dimension
    T1b   More than 0.5 cm but not more than 1 cm in greatest dimension
    T1c   More than 1 cm but not more than 2 cm in greatest dimension
T2   Tumour more than 2 cm but not more than 5 cm in greatest dimension
T3   Tumour more than 5 cm in greatest dimension
T4   Tumour of any size with direct extension to chest wall or skin

Note: Chest wall includes ribs, intercostal muscles and serratus anterior muscle but not pectoral muscle.

    T4a   Extension to chest wall
    T4b   Oedema (including peau d'orange), or ulceration of the skin of the breast, or satellite skin nodules confined to the same breast
    T4c   Both 4a and 4b, above
    T4d   Inflammatory carcinoma

Notes: Inflammatory carcinoma of the breast is characterized by diffuse, brawny induration of the skin with an erysipeloid edge, usually with no underlying palpable mass. If the skin biopsy is negative and there is no localized, measurable primary cancer, the T category is pTX when pathologically staging a clinical inflammatory carcinoma (T4d).

When classifying pT the tumour size is a measurement of the *invasive* component. If there is a large in situ component (e.g. 4 cm) and a small invasive component (e.g. 0.5 cm) the tumour is coded pT1a.

Dimpling of the skin, nipple retraction or other skin changes, except those in T4, may occur in T1, T2 or T3 without affecting the classification.

N – Regional Lymph Nodes

NX   Regional lymph nodes cannot be assessed (e.g. previously removed)

N0   No regional lymph node metastasis

N1   Metastasis to movable ipsilateral axillary node(s)

N2   Metastasis to ipsilateral axillary node(s) fixed to one another or to other structures

N3   Metastasis to ipsilateral internal mammary lymph node(s)

M – Distant Metastasis

MX   Presence of distant metastasis cannot be assessed

M0   No distant metastasis

M1   Distant metastasis (includes metastasis to supraclavicular lymph nodes)

The category M1 may be further specified according to the following notation:

Pulmonary	PUL	Bone marrow	MAR
Osseous	OSS	Pleura	PLE
Hepatic	HEP	Peritoneum	PER
Brain	BRA	Skin	SKI
Lymph nodes	LYM	Other	OTH

pTNM Pathological Classification

pT – Primary Tumour

The pathological classification requires the examination of the primary carcinoma with no gross tumour at the margins of resection. A case can be classified pT if there is only microscopic tumour in a margin.

The pT categories correspond to the T categories.

pN – Regional Lymph Nodes

The pathological classification requires the resection and examination of at least the low axillary lymph nodes (level I) (see p. 94). Such a resection will ordinarily include 6 or more lymph nodes.

pNX Regional lymph nodes cannot be assessed (not removed for study or previously removed)

pN0 No regional lymph node metastasis

pN1 Metastasis to movable ipsilateral axillary node(s)

    pN1a Only micrometastasis (none larger than 0.2 cm)

    pN1b Metastasis to lymph node(s), any larger than 0,2 cm

        pN1bi Metastasis in 1 to 3 lymph nodes, any more than 0.2 cm and all less than 2.0 cm in greatest dimension

        pN1bii Metastasis to 4 or more lymph nodes, any more than 0.2 cm and all less than 2.0 cm in greatest dimension

        pN1biii Extension of tumor beyond the capsule of a lymph node metastasis less than 2.0 cm in greatest dimension

        pN1biv Metastasis to a lymph node 2.0 cm or more in greatest dimension

pN2 Metastasis to ipsilateral axillary lymph nodes that are fixed to one another or to other structures

pN3 Metastasis to ipsilateral internal mammary lymph node(s)

pM – Distant Metastasis

The pM categories correspond to the M categories.

G Histopathological Grading

GX   Grade of differentiation cannot be assessed
G1   Well differentiated
G2   Moderately differentiated
G3   Poorly differentiated
G4   Undifferentiated

R Classification

The absence or presence of residual tumour after treatment may
be described by the symbol R:
RX   Presence of residual tumour cannot be assessed
R0   No residual tumour
T1   Microscopic residual tumour
R2   Macroscopic residual tumour

Stage Grouping

Stage 0	Tis	N0	M0
Stage I	T1	N0	M0
Stage IIA	T0	N1	M0
	T1	N1[1]	M0
	T2	N0	M0
Stage IIB	T2	N1	M0
	T3	N0	M0
Stage IIIA	T0	N2	M0
	T1	N2	M0
	T2	N2	M0
	T3	N1, N2	M0
Stage IIIB	T4	Any N	M0
	Any T	N3	M0
Stage IV	Any T	Any N	M1

Note: [1] The prognosis of patients with pN1a is similar to that of patients with
pN0.

Summary

Breast				
Tis		In situ		
T1		≤ 2 cm		
	T1a	≤ 0.5 cm		
	T1b	> 0.5 to 1 cm		
	T1c	> 1 to 2 cm		
T2		> 2 to 5 cm		
T3		> 5 cm		
T4		Chest wall/skin		
	T4a	Chest wall		
	T4b	Skin oedema/ulceration, satellite skin nodules		
	T4c	Both 4a and 4b		
	T4d	Inflammatory carcinoma		
N1		Movable axillary	pN1	
			pN1a	Micrometastasis only ≤ 0.2 cm
			pN1b	Gross metastasis
				i 1–3 nodes/ > 0.2 to < 2 cm
				ii ≥ 4 nodes/ > 0.2 to < 2 cm
				iii through capsule/ < 2 cm
				iv ≥ 2 cm
N2		Fixed axillary	pN2	
N3		Internal mammary	pN3	

GYNAECOLOGICAL TUMOURS

Introductory Notes

The following sites are included:

Cervix uteri
Corpus uteri
Ovary
Vagina
Vulva

Cervix uteri and corpus uteri were amongst the first sites to be classified by the TNM system. The "League of Nations" stages for carcinoma of the cervix have been used with minor modifications for nearly 50 years and because these are accepted by the Fédération Internationale de Gynécologie et d'Obstétrique (FIGO), the TNM categories have been defined to correspond to the FIGO stages. Some amendments have been made in collaboration with FIGO and the classifications now published have the approval of FIGO, UICC and the national TNM committees including AJCC.

Each site is described under the following headings:

Rules for classification with the procedures for assessing the T, N and M categories. Additional methods may be used when they enhance the accuracy of appraisal before treatment
Anatomical subsites
Definition of the regional lymph nodes
TNM Clinical classification
pTNM Pathological classification
Stage grouping
Summary

Additional Descriptors

When appropriate, the y symbol, the r symbol and the C-factor category may be added (see p. 9).

Distant Metastasis

The definitions of the M categories for all gynaecological sites are:

M – Distant Metastasis

MX   Presence of distant metastasis cannot be assessed
M0   No distant metastasis
M1   Distant metastasis
  The categories M1 and pM1 may be further specified according to the following notation:

Pulmonary	PUL	Bone Marrow	MAR
Osseous	OSS	Pleura	PLE
Hepatic	HEP	Peritoneum	PER
Brain	BRA	Skin	SKI
Lymph nodes	LYM	Other	OTH

Histopathological Grading

The definitions of the G categories apply to cervix, vagina and vulva. These are:

G – Histopathological Grading

GX   Grade of differentiation cannot be assessed
G1   Well differentiated
G2   Moderately differentiated
G3   Poorly differentiated
G4   Undifferentiated

R Classification

The absence or presence of residual tumour after treatment may
be described by the symbol R. The definitions of the R classification apply to all gynaecological tumours. These are:

RX   Presence of residual tumour cannot be assessed
R0   No residual tumour
R1   Microscopic residual tumour
R2   Macroscopic residual tumour

Cervix Uteri (ICD-0 180)

The definitions of the T categories correspond to the several stages accepted by FIGO. Both systems are included for comparison.

Rules for Classification

The classification applies only to carcinoma. There should be histological confirmation of the disease.

The following are the procedures for assessing the T, N and M categories:

T categories   Physical examination, cystoscopy[1] and imaging including urography.

N categories   Physical examination and imaging including urography and lymphography.

M categories   Physical examination and imaging.

Note: [1] Cystoscopy not required for Tis.

Anatomical Subsites

1. Endocervix (180.0)
2. Exocervix (180.1)

Regional Lymph Nodes

The regional lymph nodes are the paracervical, parametrial, hypogastric (obturator), common, internal and external iliac, presacral and sacral nodes.

TNM Clinical Classification

T – Primary Tumour

TNM categories	FIGO stages	
TX		Primary tumour cannot be assessed
T0		No evidence of primary tumour
Tis	0	Carcinoma in situ
T1	I	Cervical carcinoma confined to uterus (extension to corpus should be disregarded)
T1a	Ia	Preclinical invasive carcinoma, diagnosed by microscopy only
T1a1	Ia1	Minimal microscopic stromal invasion
T1a2	Ia2	Tumour with invasive component 5 mm or less in depth, taken from the base of the epithelium, *and* 7 mm or less in horizontal spread
T1b	Ib	Tumour larger than T1a2
T2	II	Cervical carcinoma invades beyond uterus but not to pelvic wall or to lower third of the vagina
T2a	IIa	Without parametrial invasion
T2b	IIb	With parametrial invasion
T3	III	Cervical carcinoma extends to pelvic wall and/or involves the lower third of the vagina and/or causes hydronephrosis or non-functioning kidney

TNM categories	FIGO stages	
T3a	IIIa	Tumour involves lower third of the vagina, no extension to pelvic wall
T3b	IIIb	Tumour extends to pelvic wall and/or causes hydronephrosis or non-functioning kidney
T4	IVa	Tumour invades *mucosa* of bladder or rectum and/or extends beyond true pelvis
		Note: The presence of bullous oedema is not sufficient evidence to classify a tumour T4.
M1	IVb	Distant metastasis

N – Regional Lymph Nodes

NX   Regional lymph nodes cannot be assessed
N0   No regional lymph node metastasis
N1   Regional lymph node metastasis

M – Distant Metastasis

See definitions p. 102.

pTNM Pathological Classification

The pT, pN and pM categories correspond to the T, N and M categories.

G Histopathological Grading

See definitions p. 102.

Stage Grouping

Stage 0	Tis	N0	M0
Stage IA	T1a	N0	M0
Stage IB	T1b	N0	M0
Stage IIA	T2a	N0	M0
Stage IIB	T2b	N0	M0
Stage IIIA	T3a	N0	M0
Stage IIIB	T1	N1	M0
	T2	N1	M0
	T3a	N1	M0
	T3b	Any N	M0
Stage IVA	T4	Any N	M0
Stage IVB	Any T	Any N	M1

Summary

TNM			Cervix uteri	*FIGO*	
Tis			In situ	0	
T1			Confined to uterus Diag-	I	
	T1a		nosed only by microscopy	Ia	
		T1a1	Minimal stromal invasion		Ia1
		T1a2	Depth ≤ 5 mm, horizontal spread ≤ 7 mm		Ia2
	T1b		Lesions greater than T1a2	Ib	
T2			Beyond uterus but not pelvic wall or lower third vagina	II	
	T2a		No parametrium	IIa	
	T2b		Parametrium	IIb	
T3			Lower third vagina/pelvic wall/hydronephrosis	III	
	T3a		Lower third vagina	IIIa	
	T3b		Pelvic wall/hydronephrosis	IIIb	
T4			Mucosa of bladder/rectum/ beyond true pelvis	IVa	
M1			Distant metastasis	IVb	

Corpus Uteri (ICD-O 182)

The definitions of the T categories correspond to the several stages accepted by FIGO. Both systems are included for comparison.

Rules for Classification

The classification applies only to carcinoma. There should be histological verification and grading of the tumour. The diagnosis should be based on examination of specimens taken by fractional curettage.

The following are the procedures for assessing the T, N and M categories:

T categories	Physical examination and imaging including urography and cystoscopy
N categories	Physical examination and imaging including urography
M categories	Physical examination and imaging

Anatomical Subsites

1. Corpus uteri (182.0)
2. Isthmus uteri (182.1)

Regional Lymph Nodes

The regional lymph nodes are the hypogastric (obturator), common, internal and external iliac, parametrial and sacral nodes.

TNM Clinical Classification

T – Primary Tumour

TNM categories	FIGO stages	
TX		Primary tumour cannot be assessed
T0		No evidence of primary tumour
Tis	0	Carcinoma in situ
T1	I	Tumour confined to corpus
T1a	Ia	Uterine cavity 8 cm or less in length
T1b	Ib	Uterine cavity more than 8 cm in length
T2	II	Tumour invades cervix but does not extend beyond uterus
T3	III	Tumour extends beyond uterus but not outside true pelvis
T4	IVa	Tumour invades *mucosa* of bladder or rectum and/or extends beyond the true pelvis **Note:** The presence of bullous oedema is not sufficient evidence to classify a tumour T4.
M1	IVb	Distant metastasis

Note: FIGO stages are further subdivided by histological grade:
    G1   Well differentiated
    G2   Moderately differentiated
    G3–4 Poorly differentiated/undifferentiated

N – Regional Lymph Nodes

NX   Regional lymph nodes cannot be assessed
N0   No regional lymph node metastasis
N1   Regional lymph node metastasis

M – Distant Metastasis

See definitions p. 102.

pTNM Pathological Classification

The pT, pN and pM categories correspond to the T, N and M categories.

Stage Grouping

Stage 0	Tis	N0	M0
Stage IA	T1a	N0	M0
Stage IB	T1b	N0	M0
Stage II	T2	N0	M0
Stage III	T1	N1	M0
	T2	N1	M0
	T3	Any N	M0
Stage IVA	T4	Any N	M0
Stage IVB	Any T	Any N	M1

Summary

TNM		Corpus uteri	FIGO	
Tis		In situ	0	
T1		Confined to corpus	I	
	T1a	Cavity ≤ 8 cm		Ia
	T1b	Cavity > 8 cm		Ib
T2		Extension to cervix	II	
T3		Extension beyond uterus/within true pelvis	III	
T4		Extension to mucosa of bladder/rectum/beyond true pelvis	IVa	
M1		Distant metastasis	IVb	

Ovary (ICD-O 183.0)

The definitions of the T categories correspond to the several stages accepted by FIGO. Both systems are included for comparison.

Rules for Classification

There should be histological confirmation of the disease to permit division of cases by histological type. In accordance with FIGO a simplified version of the WHO histological typing (1973, publication no. 9) is recommended. The degree of differentiation (grade) should be recorded.

The following are the procedures for assessing the T, N and M categories:

T categories   Physical examination, imaging, laparoscopy and/or surgical exploration

N categories   Physical examination, imaging, laparoscopy and/or surgical exploration

M categories   Physical examination, imaging, laparoscopy and/or surgical exploration

Regional Lymph Nodes

The regional lymph nodes are the hypogastric (obturator), common iliac, external iliac, lateral sacral, para-aortic and inguinal nodes.

TNM Clinical Classification

T – Primary Tumour

TNM categories		FIGO stages	
TX			Primary tumour cannot be assessed
T0			No evidence of primary tumour
T1		I	Tumour limited to ovaries
	T1a	Ia	Tumour limited to one ovary; capsule intact, no tumour on ovarian surface
	T1b	Ib	Tumour limited to both ovaries; capsules intact, no tumour on ovarian surface
	T1c	Ic	Tumour limited to one or both ovaries with any of the following: capsule ruptured, tumour on ovarian surface, malignant cells in ascites or peritoneal washing
T2		II	Tumour involves one or both ovaries with pelvic extension
	T2a	IIa	Extension and/or implants on uterus and/or tube(s)
	T2b	IIb	Extension to other pelvic tissues
	T2c	IIc	Pelvic extension (2a or 2b) with malignant cells in ascites or peritoneal washing
T3 and/or N1		III	Tumour involves one or both ovaries with microscopically confirmed peritoneal metastasis outside the pelvis and/or regional lymph node metastasis
	T3a	IIIa	Microscopic peritoneal metastasis beyond pelvis
	T3b	IIIb	Macroscopic peritoneal metastasis beyond pelvis 2 cm or less in greatest dimension

TNM categories	FIGO stages	
T3c and/or N1	IIIc	Peritoneal metastasis beyond pelvis more than 2 cm in greatest dimension and/or regional lymph node metastasis
M1	IV	Distant metastasis (excludes peritoneal metastasis)

Note: Liver capsule metastasis is T3/stage III, liver parenchymal metastasis M1/stage IV. Pleural effusion must have positive cytology for M1/stage IV.

N - Regional Lymph Nodes

NX   Regional lymph nodes cannot be assessed
N0   No regional lymph node metastasis
N1   Regional lymph node metastasis

M - Distant Metastasis

See p. 102.

pTNM Pathological Classification

The pT, pN and pM categories correspond to the T, N and M categories.

G Histopathological Grading

GX   Grade cannot be assessed
GB   Borderline malignancy
G1   Well differentiated
G2   Moderately differentiated
G3-4 Poorly differentiated or undifferentiated

Stage Grouping

Stage IA	T1a	N0	M0
Stage IB	T1b	N0	M0
Stage IC	T1c	N0	M0
Stage IIA	T2a	N0	M0
Stage IIB	T2b	N0	M0
Stage IIC	T2c	N0	M0
Stage IIIA	T3a	N0	M0
Stage IIIB	T3b	N0	M0
Stage IIIC	T3c	N0	M0
	Any T	N1	M0
Stage IV	Any T	Any N	M1

Summary

TNM		Ovary	FIGO
T1		Limited to ovaries	I
	T1a	One ovary, capsule intact	Ia
	T1b	Both ovaries, capsule intact	Ib
	T1c	Capsule ruptured, tumour on surface, malignant cells in ascites or peritoneal washings	Ic
T2		Pelvic extension	II
	T2a	Uterus, tube(s)	IIa
	T2b	Other pelvic tissues	IIb
	T2c	Malignant cells in ascites or peritoneal washings	IIc
T3 and/ or N1		Peritoneal metastasis beyond pelvis and/or regional lymph node metastasis	III
	T3a	Microscopic peritoneal metastasis	IIIa
	T3b	Macroscopic peritoneal metastasis ≤ 2 cm	IIIb
	T3c and/or N1	Peritoneal metastasis > 2 cm and/or regional lymph node metastasis	IIIc
M1		Distant metastasis (excludes peritoneal metastasis)	IV

Vagina (ICD-O 184.0)

The definitions of the T categories correspond to the several stages accepted by FIGO. Both systems are included for comparison.

Rules for Classification

The classification applies to primary carcinoma only. Tumours present in the vagina as secondary growths from either genital or extragenital sites should be excluded. A tumour that has extended to the portio and reached the external os should be classified as carcinoma of the cervix. A tumour involving the vulva should be classified as carcinoma of the vulva. There should be histological confirmation of the disease.

The following are the procedures for assessing the T, N and M categories:

T categories   Physical examination, endoscopy and imaging
N categories   Physical examination and imaging
M categories   Physical examination and imaging

Regional Lymph Nodes

Upper two-thirds of vagina: the pelvic nodes.
Lower third of vagina: the inguinal nodes.

TNM Clinical Classification

T – Primary Tumour

TNM categories	FIGO stages	
TX		Primary tumour cannot be assessed
T0		No evidence of primary tumour
Tis	0	Carcinoma in situ
T1	I	Tumour confined to vagina
T2	II	Tumour invades paravaginal tissues but not to pelvic wall
T3	III	Tumour extends to pelvic wall
T4	IVa	Tumour invades *mucosa* of bladder or rectum and/or extends beyond the true pelvis
		Note: The presence of bullous oedema is not sufficient evidence to classify a tumour T4.
M1	IVb	Distant metastasis

N – Regional Lymph Nodes

NX   Regional lymph nodes cannot be assessed
N0   No regional lymph node metastasis

Upper Two-Thirds of Vagina

N1   Pelvic lymph node metastasis

Lower Third of Vagina

N1   Unilateral inguinal lymph node metastasis
N2   Bilateral inguinal lymph node metastasis

M – Distant Metastasis

See definitions p. 102.

pTNM Pathological Classification

The pT, pN and pM categories correspond to the T, N and M categories.

G Histopathological Grading

See definitions p. 102.

Stage Grouping

Stage 0	Tis	N0	M0
Stage I	T1	N0	M0
Stage II	T2	N0	M0
Stage III	T1	N1	M0
	T2	N1	M0
	T3	N0, N1	M0
Stage IVA	T1	N2	M0
	T2	N2	M0
	T3	N2	M0
	T4	Any N	M0
Stage IVB	Any T	Any N	M1

Summary

TNM	Vagina	*FIGO*
T1	Vagina wall	I
T2	Paravaginal tissue not to pelvic wall	II
T3	Extends to pelvic wall	III
T4	Mucosa of bladder/rectum, beyond pelvis	IVa
Upper two-thirds		
N1	Pelvic	III
Lower third		
N1	Unilateral inguinal	IVa
N2	Bilateral inguinal	IVa
M1	Distant metastasis	IVb

Vulva (ICD-O 184.1–4)

The classification for carcinomas of the vulva is taken directly from FIGO. While it is not consistent with the principles of the TNM used for other anatomical sites, it is accepted in the spirit of unanimity in order to facilitate comparison of data throughout the world.

Rules for Classification

The classification applies only to primary carcinoma of the vulva. There should be histological confirmation of the disease. A carcinoma of the vulva that has extended to the vagina should be classified as carcinoma of the vulva.

The following are the procedures for assessing the T, N and M categories:

T categories	Physical examination, endoscopy and imaging
N categories	Physical examination and imaging
M categories	Physical examination and imaging

Regional Lymph Nodes

The regional lymph nodes are the femoral, inguinal, external and internal iliac (hypogastric) nodes.

TNM Clinical Classification (FIGO)

T – Primary Tumour

TX	Primary tumour cannot be assessed
T0	No evidence of primary tumour
Tis	Carcinoma in situ

T1   Tumour confined to vulva, 2 cm or less in greatest dimension

T2   Tumour confined to vulva, more than 2 cm in greatest dimension

T3   Tumour invades any of the following: urethra, vagina, perineum, anus

T4   Tumour invades any of the following: bladder mucosa, upper part of urethral mucosa, rectal mucosa or tumour fixed to the bone

N – Regional Lymph Nodes

NX   Regional lymph nodes cannot be assessed

N0   No nodes palpable

N1   Nodes palpable in either groin, not enlarged, mobile (not clinically suspicious of neoplasm)

N2   Nodes palpable in either groin, enlarged, firm and mobile (clinically suspicious of neoplasm)

N3   Fixed or ulcerated nodes

M – Distant Metastasis

MX   Presence of distant metastasis cannot be assessed

M0   No clinical metastasis

M1a   Palpable deep pelvic lymph nodes

M1b   Other distant metastasis

G Histopathological Grading

See definitions p. 102.

Clinical Stage Grouping

Stage 0	Tis	N0	M0
Stage I	T1	N0, N1	M0
Stage II	T2	N0, N1	M0
Stage III	T1	N2	M0
	T2	N2	M0
	T3	N0, N1, N2	M0
Stage IV	T4	Any N	M0
	Any T	N3	M0
	Any T	Any N	M1a, 1b

Summary

TNM	Vulva	*FIGO*
T1	$\leqslant 2$ cm	I
T2	> 2 cm	II
T3	Urethra/vagina/perineum/anus	III
T4	Bladder mucosa/upper urethra mucosa/rectum mucosa/pelvic bone	IV
N1	Palpable, not clinically suspicious of neoplasm	I or II
N2	Palpable, clinically suspicious of neoplasm	III
N3	Fixed or ulcerated	IV
M1a	Palpable deep pelvic nodes	IV
M1b	Other distant metastasis	IV

UROLOGICAL TUMOURS

Introductory Notes

The following sites are included:

Prostate
Testis
Penis
Urinary bladder
Kidney
Renal pelvis and ureter
Urethra

Each site is described under the following headings:

Rules for classification with the procedures for assessing the T, N
and M categories. Additional methods may be used when they
enhance the accuracy of appraisal before treatment
Anatomical sites and subsites where appropriate
Definition of the regional lymph nodes
TNM Clinical classification
pTNM Pathological classification
G Histopathological grading where applicable
Stage grouping
Summary

Additional Descriptors

When appropriate, the y symbol, the r symbol and the C-factor
category may be added (see p. 9).

The suffix (m) should be added to the appropriate T category
to indicate multiple lesions.

Regional Lymph Nodes

The definitions of the N categories apply to all urological sites except penis. These are:

N – Regional Lymph Nodes

NX   Regional lymph nodes cannot be assessed
N0   No regional lymph node metastasis
N1   Metastasis in a single lymph node 2 cm or less in greatest dimension
N2   Metastasis in a single lymph node more than 2 cm but not more than 5 cm in greatest dimension, or multiple lymph nodes, none more than 5 cm in greatest dimension
N3   Metastasis in a lymph node more than 5 cm in greatest dimension

Distant Metastasis

The definitions of the M categories for all urological tumours are:

M – Distant Metastasis

MX   Presence of distant metastasis cannot be assessed
M0   No distant metastasis
M1   Distant metastasis
The categories M1 and pM1 may be further specified according to the following notation:

Pulmonary	PUL	Bone marrow	MAR
Osseous	OSS	Pleura	PLE
Hepatic	HEP	Peritoneum	PER
Brain	BRA	Skin	SKI
Lymph nodes	LYM	Other	OTH

Histopathological Grading

The definitions of the G categories apply to all urological sites except prostate and testis. These are:

G – Histopathological Grading

GX   Grade of differentiation cannot be assessed
G1   Well differentiated
G2   Moderately differentiated
G3–4 Poorly differentiated/undifferentiated

R Classification

The absence or presence of residual tumour after treatment may be described by the symbol R. The definitions of the R classification apply to all urological sites. These are:
RX   Presence of residual tumour cannot be assessed
R0   No residual tumour
R1   Microscopic residual tumour
R2   Macroscopic residual tumour

Prostate (ICD-O 185)

Rules for Classification

The classification applies only to carcinoma. There should be histological confirmation of the disease.

The following are the procedures for assessment of the T, N and M categories:

T categories Physical examination, imaging, endoscopy and biopsy
N categories Physical examination and imaging
M categories Physical examination, imaging, skeletal studies and biochemical tests

Regional Lymph Nodes

The regional lymph nodes are the nodes of the true pelvis which essentially are the pelvic nodes below the bifurcation of the common iliac arteries. Laterality does not affect the N classification.

TNM Clinical Classification

T – Primary Tumour

TX   Primary tumour cannot be assessed
T0   No evidence of primary tumour

T1   Tumour is incidental histological finding
       T1a   3 or fewer microscopic foci of carcinoma
       T1b   More than 3 microscopic foci of carcinoma
T2   Tumour present clinically or grossly, limited to the gland
       T2a   Tumour 1.5 cm or less in greatest dimension with normal tissue on at least three sides

T2b Tumour more than 1.5 cm in greatest dimension or in more than one lobe

T3 Tumour invades into the prostatic apex or into or beyond the prostatic capsule or bladder neck or seminal vesical, but is not fixed

T4 Tumour is fixed or invades adjacent structures other than those listed in T3

N – Regional Lymph Nodes

See definitions p. 122.

M – Distant Metastasis

See definitions p. 122.

pTNM Pathological Classification

The pT, pN and pM categories correspond to the T, N and M categories.

G Histopathological Grading

GX Grade of differentiation cannot be assessed
G1 Well differentiated, slight anaplasia
G2 Moderately differentiated, moderate anaplasia
G3–4 Poorly differentiated-undifferentiated, marked anaplasia

Stage Grouping

Stage 0	T1a	N0	M0	G1
	T2a	N0	M0	G1
Stage I	T1a	N0	M0	G2, 3-4
	T2a	N0	M0	G2, 3-4
Stage II	T1b	N0	M0	Any G
	T2b	N0	M0	Any G
Stage III	T3	N0	M0	Any G
Stage IV	T4	N0	M0	Any G
	Any T	N1, N2, N3	M0	Any G
	Any T	Any N	M1	Any G

Summary

Prostate	
T1	Incidental
T1a	$\leqslant$ 3 foci
T1b	> 3 foci
T2	Clinically or grossly, limited to gland
T2a	$\leqslant$ 1.5 cm
T2b	> 1.5 cm/ > one lobe
T3	Invades prostatic apex/beyond capsule/bladder neck/seminal vesical/not fixed
T4	Fixed or invades other adjacent structures
N1	Single $\leqslant$ 2 cm
N2	Single > 2 cm $\leqslant$ 5 cm, multiple $\leqslant$ 5 cm
N3	> 5 cm

Testis (ICD-O 186)

Rules for Classification

Testis refers to the body of the testis and excludes the epididymis. There should be histological confirmation of the disease to permit division of cases by histological type. Histopathological grading is not applicable for testis cancer. Malignant lymphoma is excluded.

The following are the procedure for assessment of the N and M categories:

N categories   Physical examination and imaging
M categories   Physical examination, imaging and biochemical tests

Regional Lymph Nodes

The regional lymph nodes are the abdominal para-aortic nodes and paracaval nodes, the intrapelvic nodes and the inguinal nodes after scrotal or inguinal surgery. Laterality does not affect the N classification.

TNM Clinical Classification

T – Primary Tumour

The extent of primary tumour is classified after radical orchiectomy, see pT. In the absence of radical orchiectomy TX is used.

N – Regional Lymph Nodes

See definitions p. 122.

M – Distant Metastasis

See definitions p. 122.

pTNM Pathological Classification

pT – Primary Tumour

pTX   Primary tumour cannot be assessed (in the absence of radical orchi-
       ectomy TX is used)
pT0   Histological scar or no evidence of primary tumour
pTis   Intratubular tumour: preinvasive cancer

pT1   Tumour limited to testis, including rete testis
pT2   Tumour invades beyond tunica albuginea or into epididy-
       mis
pT3   Tumour invades spermatic cord
pT4   Tumour invades scrotum

pN – Regional Lymph Nodes

The pN categories correspond to the N categories.

pM – Distant Metastasis

The pM categories correspond to the M categories.

Stage Grouping

Stage 0	pTis	N0	M0
Stage I	pT1	N0	M0
	pT2	N0	M0
Stage II	pT3	N0	M0
	pT4	N0	M0
Stage III	Any pT	N1	M0
Stage IV	Any pT	N2, N3	M0
	Any pT	Any N	M1

Summary

Testis	
pTis	Intratubular
pT1	Testis and rete testis
pT2	Beyond tunica albuginea or into epididymis
pT3	Spermatic cord
pT4	Scrotum
N1	Single $\leqslant 2$ cm
N2	Single > 2 cm $\leqslant 5$ cm, multiple $\leqslant 5$ cm
N3	> 5 cm

Penis (ICD-O 187)

Rules for Classification

The classification applies only to carcinoma. There should be histological confirmation of the disease.

The following are the procedures for assessment of the T, N and M categories:

T categories   Physical examination and endoscopy
N categories   Physical examination and imaging
M categories   Physical examination and imaging

Anatomical Subsites

1. Preputium or prepuce (187.1)
2. Glans penis (187.2)
3. Shaft of penis (187.3)

Regional Lymph Nodes

The regional lymph nodes are the superficial and deep inguinal and the pelvic nodes.

TNM Clinical Classification

T – Primary Tumour

TX   Primary tumour cannot be assessed
T0   No evidence of primary tumour
Tis   Carcinoma in situ
Ta   Non-invasive verrucous carcinoma

T1   Tumour invades subepithelial connective tissue
T2   Tumour invades corpus spongiosum or cavernosum
T3   Tumour invades urethra or prostate
T4   Tumour invades other adjacent structures

N – Regional Lymph Nodes

NX   Regional lymph nodes cannot be assessed
N0   No regional lymph node metastasis
N1   Metastasis in a single superficial inguinal lymph node
N2   Metastasis in multiple or bilateral superficial inguinal lymph nodes
N3   Metastasis in deep inguinal or pelvic lymph node(s), unilateral or bilateral

M – Distant Metastasis

See definitions p. 122.

pTNM Pathological Classification

The pT, pN and pM categories correspond to the T, N and M categories.

G Histopathological Grading

See definitions p. 122.

Stage Grouping

Stage 0	Tis	N0	M0
	Ta	N0	M0
Stage I	T1	N0	M0
Stage II	T1	N1	M0
	T2	N0, N1	M0
Stage III	T1	N2	M0
	T2	N2	M0
	T3	N0, N1, N2	M0
Stage IV	T4	Any N	M0
	Any T	N3	M0
	Any T	Any N	M1

Summary

Penis	
Tis	In situ
Ta	Non-invasive verrucous carcinoma
T1	Subepithelial connective tissue
T2	Corpus spongiosum, cavernosum
T3	Urethra, prostate
T4	Other adjacent structures
N1	One superficial inguinal
N2	Multiple or bilateral superficial inguinal
N3	Deep inguinal or pelvic

Urinary Bladder (ICD-O 188)

Rules for Classification

The classification applies only to carcinoma. Papilloma is excluded. There should be histological or cytological confirmation of the disease.

The following are the procedures for assessment of the T, N and M categories:

T categories   Physical examination, imaging, endoscopy and biopsy
N categories   Physical examination and imaging
M categories   Physical examination and imaging

Regional Lymph Nodes

The regional lymph nodes are the nodes of the true pelvis which essentially are the pelvic nodes below the bifurcation of the common iliac arteries. Laterality does not affect the N classification.

TNM Clinical Classification

T – Primary Tumour

The suffix (m) should be added to the appropriate T category to indicate multiple tumours. The suffix (is) may be added to any T to indicate presence of associated carcinoma in situ.

TX   Primary tumour cannot be assessed
T0   No evidence of primary tumour
Tis   Carcinoma in situ: "flat tumour"
  Ta   Non-invasive papillary carcinoma

T1   Tumour invades subepithelial connective tissue
T2   Tumour invades superficial muscle (inner half)
T3   Tumour invades deep muscle or perivesical fat
    T3a   Tumour invades deep muscle (outer half)
    T3b   Tumour invades perivesical fat
T4   Tumour invades any of the following: prostate, uterus, vagina, pelvic wall, abdominal wall

Note: If pathology report does not specify that tumour invades muscle, consider as invasion of subepithelial connective tissue. If depth of muscle invasion is not specified by the surgeon, code as T2.

N – Regional Lymph Nodes

See definitions p. 122.

M – Distant Metastasis

See definitions p. 122.

pTNM Pathological Classification

The pT, pN and pM categories correspond to the T, N and M categories.

G Histopathological Grading

See definitions p. 122.

Stage Grouping

Stage 0	Tis	N0	M0
	Ta	N0	M0
Stage I	T1	N0	M0
Stage II	T2	N0	M0
Stage III	T3a	N0	M0
	T3b	N0	M0
Stage IV	T4	N0	M0
	Any T	N1, N2, N3	M0
	Any T	Any N	M1

Summary

Urinary bladder	
Tis	In situ: "flat tumour"
Ta	Papillary non-invasive
T1	Subepithelial connective tissue
T2	Superficial muscle (inner half)
T3	Deep muscle or perivesical fat
T3a	Deep muscle (outer half)
T3b	Perivesical fat
T4	Prostate, uterus, vagina, pelvic wall, abdominal wall
N1	Single ≤ 2 cm
N2	Single > 2 cm ≤ 5 cm, multiple ≤ 5 cm
N3	> 5 cm

Kidney (ICD-O 189.0)

Rules for Classification

The classification applies only to renal-cell carcinoma. Adenoma is excluded. There should be histological confirmation of the disease.

The following are the procedures for assessment of the T, N and M categories.

T categories   Physical examination and imaging
N categories   Physical examination and imaging
M categories   Physical examination and imaging

Regional Lymph Nodes

The regional lymph nodes are the hilar, abdominal para-aortic and paracaval nodes. Laterality does not affect the N categories.

TNM Clinical Classification

T – Primary Tumor

TX   Primary tumour cannot be assessed
T0   No evidence of primary tumour

T1   Tumour 2.5 cm on less in greatest dimension, limited to the kidney
T2   Tumour more than 2.5 cm in greatest dimension, limited to the kidney
T3   Tumour extends into major veins or invades adrenal gland or perinephric tissues but not beyond Gerota's fascia
    T3a   Tumour invades adrenal gland or perinephric tissues but not beyond Gerota's fascia

T3b   Tumour grossly extends into renal vein(s) or vena
        cava
T4   Tumour invades beyond Gerota's fascia

N - Regional Lymph Nodes

See definitions . 122.

M - Distant Metastasis

See definitions p. 122.

pTNM Pathological Classification

The pT, pN and pM categories correspond to the T, N and M
categories.

G Histopathological Grading

See definitions p. 123.

Stage Grouping

Stage I	T1	N0	M0
Stage II	T2	N0	M0
Stage III	T1	N1	M0
	T2	N1	M0
	T3a	N0, N1	M0
	T3b	N0, N1	M0
Stage IV	T4	Any N	M0
	Any T	N2, N3	M0
	Any T	Any N	M1

Summary

Kidney	
T1	⩽ 2.5 cm/limited to kidney
T2	> 2.5 cm/limited to kidney
T3	Into major veins or perinephric invasion
T4	Invades beyond Gerota's fascia
N1	Single ⩽ 2 cm
N2	Single > 2 cm ⩽ 5 cm, multiple ⩽ 5 cm
N3	> 5 cm

Renal Pelvis and Ureter (ICD-O 189.1, 2)

Rules for Classification

The classification applies only to carcinoma. Papilloma is excluded. There should be histological or cytological confirmation of the disease.

The following are the procedures for assessment of the T, N and M categories:

T categories Physical examination, imaging and endoscopy
M categories Physical examination and imaging
M categories Physical examination and imaging

Anatomical Sites

1. Renal pelvis (189.1)
2. Ureter (189.2)

Regional Lymph Nodes

The regional lymph nodes are the hilar, abdominal para-aortic, paracaval and intrapelvic nodes. Laterality does not effect the N classification.

TNM Clinical Classification

T – Primary Tumour

TX   Primary tumour cannot be assessed
T0   No evidence of primary tumour
Tis   Carcinoma in situ
  Ta   Papillary non-invasive carcinoma

T1   Tumour invades subepithelial connective tissue
T2   Tumour invades muscularis
T3   Tumour invades beyond muscularis into peri-ureteric or
      peripelvic fat or renal parenchyma
T4   Tumour invades adjacent organs or through the kidney
      into the perinephric fat

N – Regional Lymph Nodes

See definitions p. 122.

M – Distant Metastasis

See definitions p. 122.

pTNM Pathological Classification

The pT, pN and pM categories correspond to the T, N and M
categories.

G Histopathological Grading

See definitions p. 123.

Stage Grouping

Stage 0	Tis	N0	M0
	Ta	N0	M0
Stage I	T1	N0	M0
Stage II	T2	N0	M0
Stage III	T3	N0	M0
Stage IV	T4	N0	M0
	Any T	N1, N2, N3	M0
	Any T	Any N	M1

Summary

Renal Pelvis, Ureter	
Tis	In situ
Ta	Non-invasive papillary
T1	Subepithelial connective tissue
T2	Muscularis
T3	Beyond muscularis
T4	Adjacent organs, perinephric fat
N1	Single $\leqslant 2$ cm
N2	Single > 2 cm $\leqslant 5$ cm, multiple $\leqslant 5$ cm
N3	> 5 cm

Urethra (ICD-O 189.3)

Rules for Classification

The classification applies only to carcinoma. There should be histological or cytological confirmation of the disease.

The following are the procedures for assessment of the T, N and M categories:

T categories	Physical examination, imaging, endoscopy and biopsy
N categories	Physical examination and imaging
M categories	Physical examination and imaging

Regional Lymph Nodes

The regional lymph nodes are the inguinal and the pelvic lymph nodes. Laterality does not affect the N classification.

TNM Clinical Classification

T – Primary Tumour

TX   Primary tumour cannot be assessed
T0   No evidence of primary tumour
Tis   Carcinoma in situ
   Ta   Non-invasive papillary, polypoid, or verrucous carcinoma

T1   Tumour invades subepithelial connective tissue
T2   Tumour invades corpus spongiosum or prostate or peri-urethral muscle
T3   Tumour invades corpus cavernosum or beyond prostatic capsule or anterior vagina or bladder neck
T4   Tumour invades other adjacent organs

N – Regional Lymph Nodes

See definitions p. 122.

M – Distant Metastasis

See definitions p. 122.

pTNM Pathological Classification

The pT, pN and pM categories correspond to the T, N and M categories.

G Histopathological Grading

See definitions p. 123.

Stage Grouping

Stage 0	Tis	N0	M0
	Ta	N0	M0
Stage I	T1	N0	M0
Stage II	T2	N0	M0
Stage III	T1	N1	M0
	T2	N1	M0
	T3	N0, N1	M0
Stage IV	T4	N0, N1	M0
	Any T	N2, N3	M0
	Any T	Any N	M1

Summary

Urethra	
Tis	In situ
Ta	Non-invasive papillary, polypoid or verrucous
T1	Subepithelial connective tissue
T2	Corpus spongiosum, prostate, periurethral muscle
T3	Corpus cavernosum, beyond prostatic capsule, anterior vagina, bladder neck
T4	Other adjacent organs
N1	Single $\leqslant 2$ cm
N2	Single > 2 cm $\leqslant 5$ cm, multiple $\leqslant 5$ cm
N3	> 5 cm

OPHTHALMIC TUMOURS

Introductory Notes

Tumours of the eye and its adnexa are a disparate group including carcinoma, melanoma, sarcoma and retinoblastoma. For clinical convenience they should be classified in one section.

Tumours in the following sites are classified:

Eyelid
Conjunctiva
Uvea
Retina
Orbit
Lacrimal gland

For histological nomenclature and diagnostic criteria, reference to the WHO classification (International Histological Classification of Tumours, No. 24, WHO, Geneva 1980) is recommended.

Each tumor type is described under the following headings:

Rules for classification with the procedures for assessing the T, N and M categories
Anatomical sites where appropriate
Definition of regional lymph nodes
TNM Clinical classification
pTNM Pathological classification
G Histopathological grading where applicable
Stage grouping where applicable
Summary

Additional Descriptors

When appropriate, the y symbol, the r symbol and the C-factor category may be added (see p. 9).

Regional Lymph Nodes

The definitions of the N categories for ophthalmic tumours excluding melonoma of eyelid are:

N – Regional Lymph Nodes

NX   Regional lymph nodes cannot be assessed
N0   No regional lymph node metastasis
N1   Regional lymph node metastasis

Distant Metastasis

The definitions of the M categories for ophthalmic tumours excluding melanoma of eyelid are:

M – Distant Metastasis

MX   Presence of distant metastasis cannot be assessed
M0   No distant metastasis
M1   Distant metastasis
     The categories M1 and pM1 may be further specified according to the following notation:

Pulmonary	PUL	Bone marrow	MAR
Osseous	OSS	Pleura	PLE
Hepatic	HEP	Peritoneum	PER
Brain	BRA	Skin	SKI
Lymph nodes	LYM	Other	OTH

Histopathological Grading

The following definitions of the G categories apply to carcinoma of eyelid and conjunctiva and sarcoma of orbit. These are:

G – Histopathological Grading

GX   Grade of differentiation cannot be assessed
G1   Well differentiated
G2   Moderately differentiated
G3   Poorly differentiated
G4   Undifferentiated

R Classification

The absence or presence of residual tumour after treatment may be described by the symbol R. The definitions of the R classification apply to all ophthalmic tumour types. These are:

RX   Presence of residual tumour cannot be assessed
R0   No residual tumour
R1   Microscopic residual tumour
R2   Macroscopic residual tumour

Carcinoma of Eyelid (ICD-O 173.1)

Rules for Classification

There should be histological confirmation of the disease to permit division of cases by histological type, e.g. basal cell, squamous cell and sebaceous carcinoma.

The following are the procedures for assessment of the T, N and M categories:

T categories   Physical examination
N categories   Physical examination
M categories   Physical examination and imaging

Regional Lymph Nodes

The regional lymph nodes are the preauricular, submandibular and cervical lymph nodes.

TNM Clinical Classification

T – Primary Tumour

TX   Primary tumour cannot be assessed
T0   No evidence of primary tumour
Tis   Carcinoma in situ

T1   Tumour of any size, not invading the tarsal plate; or at eyelid margin 5 mm or less in greatest dimension
T2   Tumour invades tarsal plate; or at eyelid margin more than 5 mm but not more than 10 mm in greatest dimension
T3   Tumour involves full eyelid thickness; or at eyelid margin more than 10 mm in greatest dimension
T4   Tumour invades adjacent structures

N – Regional Lymph Nodes

See definitions p. 146.

M – Distant Metastasis

See definitions p. 146.

pTNM Pathological Classification

The pT, pN and pM categories correspond to the T, N and M categories.

G Histopathological Grading

See definitions p. 147.

Stage Grouping

No stage grouping in presently recommended.

Summary

Eyelid Carcinoma	
T1	Not in tarsal plate
	Lid margin: ≤ 5 mm
T2	In tarsal plate
	Lid margin: > 5 to 10 mm
T3	Full thickness
	Lid margin: > 10 mm
T4	Adjacent structures
N1	Regional

Malignant Melanoma of Eyelid (ICD-O 173.1)

Rules for Classification

The classification is identical to that of malignant melanoma of the skin (see p. 89). There should be histological confirmation of the disease.

The following are the procedures for assessment of the N and M categories:

N categories Physical examination
M categories Physical examination and imaging

Regional Lymph Nodes

The regional lymph nodes are the preauricular, submandibular and cervical lymph nodes.

TNM Clinical Classification

T – Primary Tumour

The extent of tumour is classified after axcision, see pT.

N – Regional Lymph Nodes

NX   Regional lymph nodes cannot be assessed
N0   No regional lymph node metastasis
N1   Metastasis 3 cm or less in greatest dimension in any regional lymph node(s)
N2   Metastasis more than 3 cm in greatest dimension in any regional lymph node(s) and/or in-transit metastasis
    N2a   Metastasis more than 3 cm in greatest dimension in any regional node(s)

N2b   In-transit metastasis
N2c   Both

Note: In-transit metastasis involves skin or subcutaneous tissue more than 2 cm from the primary tumour not beyond the regional lymph nodes.

M – Distant Metastasis

MX   Presence of distant metastasis cannot be assessed
M0   No distant metastasis
M1   Distant metastasis
    M1a   Metastasis in skin or subcutaneous tissue or lymph node(s) beyond the regional lymph nodes
  M1b Visceral metastasis

pTNM Pathological Classification

pT – Primary Tumour

pTX   Primary tumour cannot be assessed
pT0   No evidence of primary tumour
pTis   Melanoma in situ (Clark's level I) (atypical melanocytic hyperplasia, severe melanocytic dysplasia, not an invasive malignant lesion)

pT1   Tumour 0.75 mm or less in thickness and invades papillary dermis (Clark's level II)
pT2   Tumour more than 0.75 mm but not more than 1.5 mm in thickness and/or invades to the papillary-reticular dermal interface (Clark's level III)
pT3   Tumour more than 1.5 mm but not more than 4.0 mm in thickness and/or invades the reticular dermis (Clarks' level IV)
    pT3a   Tumour more than 1.5 mm but not more than 3.0 mm in thickness
    pT3b   Tumour more than 3.0 mm but not more than 4.0 mm in thickness
pT4   Tumour more than 4.0 mm in thickness and/or invades subcutaneous tissue (Clark's level V) and/or satellite(s) within 2 cm of the primary tumour

pT4a   Tumour more than 4.0 mm in thickness and/or
       invading subcutaneous tissue
pT4b   Satellite(s) within 2 cm of the primary tumour

Note: In case of discrepancy between tumour thickness and level, the pT
category is based on the less favourable finding.

pN - Regional Lymph Nodes

The pN categories correspond to the N categories.

pM - Distant Metastasis

The pM categories correspond to the M categories.

Stage Grouping

Stage I	pT1	N0	M0
	pT2	N0	M0
Stage II	pT3	N0	M0
Stage III	pT4	N0	M0
	Any pT	N1, N2	M0
Stage IV	Any pT	Any N	M1

Summary

Eyelid Malignant Melanoma		
pT1	≤ 0.75 mm	Level II
pT2	> 0.75 to 1.5 mm	Level III
pT3	> 1.5 to 4 mm	Level IV
pT4	> 4.0 mm/satellites	Level V
N1	Regional ≤ 3 cm	
N2	Regional > 3 cm and/or in-transit metastasis	

Carcinoma of Conjunctiva (ICD-O 190.3)

Rules for Classification

There should be histological confirmation of the disease to permit division of cases by histological type, i.e. mucoepidermoid and squamous cell carcinoma.

The following are the procedures for assessment of the T, N and M categories:

T categories Physical examination
N categories Physical examination
M categories Physical examination and imaging

Regional Lymph Nodes

The regional lymph nodes are the preauricular, submandibular and cervical nodes.

TNM Clinical Classification

T - Primary Tumour

TX   Primary tumour cannot be assessed
T0   No evidence of primary tumour
Tis   Carcinoma in situ

T1   Tumour 5 mm or less in greatest dimension
T2   Tumour more than 5 mm in greatest dimension, without invasion of adjacent structures
T3   Tumour invades adjacent structures, excluding the orbit
T4   Tumour invades the orbit

N – Regional Lymph Nodes

See definitions p. 146.

M – Distant Metastasis

See definitions p. 146.

pTNM Pathological Classification

The pT, pN and pM categories correspond to the T, N and M categories.

G Histopathological Grading

See definitions p. 147.

Stage Grouping

No stage grouping is presently recommended.

Summary

Conjunctiva Carcinoma	
T1	≤ 5 mm
T2	> 5 mm without invasion of adjacent structures
T3	Adjacent structures
T4	Orbit
N1	Regional

Malignant Melanoma of Conjunctiva
(ICD-O 190.3)

Rules for Classification

There should be histological confirmation of the disease. The tumour should be distinguished from non-tumorous pigmentation. Primary acquired melanosis should be classified under the category T0; however, in case of histological and/or cytological confirmation such cases should be listed unter G0.

The following are the procedures for assessment of T, N and M categories:

T categories   Physical examination
N categories   Physical examination
M categories   Physical examination and imaging

Regional Lymph Nodes

The regional lymph nodes are the preauricular, submandibular and cervical nodes.

TNM Clinical Classification

T – Primary Tumour

TX   Primary tumour cannot be assessed
T0   No evidence of primary tumour

T1   Tumour(s) of bulbar conjunctiva occupying one quadrant or less

T2   Tumour(s) of bulbar conjunctiva occupying more than one quadrant

T3   Tumour(s) of conjunctival fornix and/or palpebral con-
       junctiva and/or caruncle
T4   Tumour invades the eyelid, cornea and/or orbit

N - Regional Lymph Nodes

See definitions p. 146.

M - Distant Metastasis

See definitions p. 146.

pTNM Pathological Classification

pT - Primary Tumour

pTX   Primary tumour cannot be assessed
pT0   No evidence of primary tumour

pT1   Tumour(s) of the bulbar conjunctiva occupying one quad-
       rant or less *and* 2 mm or less in thickness
pT2   Tumour(s) of the bulbar conjunctiva occupying more than
       one quadrant *and* 2 mm or less in thickness
pT3   Tumour(s) of the conjunctival fornix and/or palpebral
       conjunctiva and/or caruncle or tumour of the bulbar con-
       junctiva more than 2 mm in thickness
pT4   Tumour invades the eyelid, cornea and/or orbit

pN - Regional Lymph Nodes

The pN categories correspond to the N categories.

pM - Distant Metastasis

The pM categories correspond to the M categories.

G Histopathological Grading

GX Grade cannot be assessed
G0 Primary acquired melanosis
G1 Malignant melanoma arising from a naevus
G2 Malignant melanoma arising from primary acquired mela-
    nosis
G3 Malignant melanoma arising de novo

Stage Grouping

No stage grouping is presently recommended.

Summary

Conjunctiva Malignant Melanoma			
T1	Bulbar conjunctiva ≤ 1 quadrant	pT1	T1 ≤ 2 mm thick
T2	Bulbar conjunctiva > 1 quadrant	pT2	T2 ≤ 2 mm thick
T3	Fornix, palpebral con-junctiva, caruncle	pT3	T1 or T2 > 2 mm thick and/or T3
T4	Invasion of eyelid, cor-nea and/or orbit	pT4	T4
N1	Regional	pN1	Regional

Malignant Melanoma of Uvea (ICD-O 190.0, 6)

Rules for Classification

There should be histological confirmation of the disease.

The following are the procedures for assessment of the T, N and M categories:

T categories Physical examination; additional methods such as fluorescein angiography and isotope examination may enhance the accuracy of appraisal

N categories Physical examination

M categories Physical examination and imaging

Regional Lymph Nodes

The regional lymph nodes are the preauricular, submandibular and cervical nodes.

Anatomical Sites

1. Iris (190.0)
2. Ciliary body (190.0)
3. Choroid (190.6)

TNM Clinical Classification

T – Primary Tumour

TX Primary tumour cannot be assessed
T0 No evidence of primary tumour

Iris

T1   Tumour limited to the iris
T2   Tumour involves one quadrant or less, with invasion into anterior chamber angle
T3   Tumour involves more than one quadrant, with invasion into anterior chamber angle
T4   Tumour with extraocular extension

Ciliary Body

T1   Tumour limited to the ciliary body
T2   Tumour invades into anterior chamber and/or iris
T3   Tumour invades choroid
T4   Tumour with extraocular extension

Choroid

T1   Tumour 10 mm or less in greatest dimension with an elevation 3 mm or less[1]
   T1a   Tumour 7 mm or less in greatest dimension with an elevation 2 mm or less
   T1b   Tumour more than 7 mm but not more than 10 mm in greatest dimension with an elevation more than 2 mm but not more than 3 mm
T2   Tumour more than 10 mm but not more than 15 mm in greatest dimension with an elevation more than 3 mm but not more than 5 mm[1]
T3   Tumour more than 15 mm in greatest dimension or with an elevation more than 5 mm[1]
T4   Tumour with extraocular extension

Note: 1 When dimension and elevation show a difference in classification, the highest category should be used for classification. The tumour base may be estimated in optic disc diameters (dd, average 1 dd = 1.5 mm) and the elevation in dioptries (average 3 dioptries = 1 mm); other techniques, such as ultrasonography and computerized stereometry, may provide a more accurate measurement.

N - Regional Lymph Nodes

See definitions p. 146.

M - Distant Metastasis

See definitions p. 146.

pTNM Pathological Classification

The pT, pN and pM categories correspond to the T, N and M categories.

G Histopathological Grading

GX   Grade cannot be assessed
G1   Spindle cell melanoma
G2   Mixed cell melanoma
G3   Epithelioid cell melanoma

Stage Grouping

If more than one of the uveal structures is involved, the classification of the most affected structure should be used.

Iris and Ciliary Body

Stage I	T1	N0	M0
Stage II	T2	N0	M0
Stage III	T3	N0	M0
Stage IV A	T4	N0	M0
Stage IV B	Any T	N1	M0
	Any T	Any N	M1

Choroid

Stage I A	T1 a	N0	M0
Stage I B	T1 b	N0	M0
Stage II	T2	N0	M0
Stage III	T3	N0	M0
Stage IV A	T4	N0	M0
Stage IV B	Any T	N1	M0
	Any T	Any N	M1

Summary

Uvea Malignant Melanoma	
	Iris Malignant Melanoma
T1	Iris
T2	≤ 1 quadrant with invasion into chamber angle
T3	> 1 quadrant with invasion into chamber angle
T4	Extraocular extension
	Ciliary Body Malignant Melanoma
T1	Ciliary body
T2	Anterior chamber and/or iris
T3	Choroid
T4	Extraocular extension
	Choroid Malignant Melanoma
T1	≤ 10 mm greatest dimension, ≤ 3 mm elevation
T1 a	≤ 7 mm greatest dimension, ≤ 2 mm elevation
T1 b	> 7 to 10 mm greatest dimension, > 2 to 3 mm elevation
T2	> 10 to 15 mm greatest dimension, > 3 to 5 mm elevation
T3	> 15 mm greatest dimension or > 5 mm elevation
T4	Extraocular extension
	All Sites
N1	Regional

Retinoblastoma (ICD-O 190.5)

Rules for Classification

In bilateral cases, each eye should be classified separately. The classification does not apply to complete spontaneous regression of the tumour. There should be histological confirmation of the disease in an enucleated eye.

The following are the procedures for assessment of the T, N and M categories:

T categories Physical examination and imaging
N categories Physical examination
M categories Physical examination and imaging; examination of bone marrow and cerebrospinal fluid may enhance the accuracy of appraisal

Regional Lymph Nodes

The regional lymph nodes are the preauricular, submandibular and cervical nodes.

TNM Clinical Classification

The extent of retinal involvement is indicated as a percentage (%).

TX   Primary tumour cannot be assessed
T0   No evidence of primary tumour

T1   Tumour(s) limited to 25% of the retina or less
T2   Tumour(s) involve(s) more than 25% but not more than 50% of the retina

T3   Tumour(s) involve(s) more than 50% of the retina and/or invade(s) beyond the retina but remain(s) intraocular

    T3a   Tumour(s) involve(s) more than 50% of the retina and/or tumour cells in the vitreous

    T3b   Tumour(s) involve(s) optic disc

    T3c   Tumour(s) involve(s) anterior chamber and/or uvea

T4   Tumour with extraocular invasion

    T4a   Tumour invades retrobulbar optic nerve

    T4b   Extraocular extension other than invasion of optic nerve

Note: The following suffixes may be added to the appropriate T categories:
- (m) to indicate multiple tumours, e.g. T2 (m)
- (f) to indicate cases with a known family history
- (d) to indicate diffuse retinal involvement without the formation of discrete masses

N – Regional Lymph Nodes

See definitions p. 146.

M – Distant Metastasis

See definitions p. 146.

pTNM Pathological Classification

pT – Primary Tumour

pTX   Primary tumour cannot be assessed
pT0   No evidence of primary tumour

pT1   Corresponds to T1
pT2   Corresponds to T2
pT3   Corresponds to T3

    pT3a   Corresponds to T3a

    pT3b   Tumour invades optic nerve as far as lamina cribrosa pT3c   Tumour in anterior chamber and/or invasion with thickening of uvea and/or intrascleral invasion

pT4   Corresponds to T4

      pT4a   Intraneural tumour beyond lamina cribrosa, but not at line of resection

      pT4b   Tumour at line of resection or other extraocular extension

pN – Regional Lymph Nodes

The pN categories correspond to the N categories.

pM – Distant Metastasis

The pM categories correspond to the M categories.

Stage Grouping

Stage I A	T1	N0	M0
Stage I B	T2	N0	M0
Stage II A	T3a	N0	M0
Stage II B	T3b	N0	M0
Stage II C	T3c	N0	M0
Stage III A	T4a	N0	M0
Stage III B	T4b	N0	M0
Stage IV	Any T	N1	M0
	Any T	Any N	M1

Summary

Retinoblastoma			
T1/pT1	≤25% of retina		
T2/pT2	>25% to 50% of retina		
T3/pT3	>50% of retina and/or intraocular beyond retina		
T3a/pT3a	>50% of retina and/or cells in vitreous		
T3b	Optic disc	pT3b	Optic nerve up to lamina cribrosa
T3c	Anterior chamber and/or uvea	pT3c	Anterior chamber and/or uvea and/or intrascleral
T4/pT4	Extraocular		
T4a	Optic nerve	pT4a	Beyond lamina cribrosa not at resection line
T4b	Other extraocular	pT4b	Other extraocular and/or at resection line
N1/pN1	Regional		

Sarcoma of Orbit (ICD-O 190.1)

Rules for Classification

The classification applies only to sarcomas of soft tissue and bone. There should be histological confirmation of the disease to permit division of cases by histological type.

The following are the procedures for assessment of the T, N and M categories:

T categories	Physical examination
N categories	Physical examination
M categories	Physical examination and imaging

Regional Lymph Nodes

The regional lymph nodes are the preauricular, submandibular and cervical lymph nodes.

TNM Clinical Classification

T – Primary Tumour

TX   Primary tumour cannot be assessed
T0   No evidence of primary tumour

T1   Tumour 15 mm or less in greatest dimension
T2   Tumour more than 15 mm in greatest dimension
T3   Tumour of any size with diffuse invasion of orbital tissues and/or bony walls
T4   Tumour invades beyond the orbit to adjacent sinuses and/or to cranium

N – Regional Lymph Nodes

See definitions p. 146.

M – Distant Metastasis

See definitions p. 146.

pTNM Pathological Classification

The pT, pN and pM categories correspond to the T, N and M categories.

Histopathological grading of the tumour should be reported and may have an effect on the staging of these tumours; however no stage grouping is presently recommended.

Summary

Sarcoma of Orbit	
T1	≤ 15 mm
T2	> 15 mm
T3	Invades orbital tissues/walls
T4	Invades beyond orbit
N1	Regional

Carcinoma of Lacrimal Gland (ICD-O 190.2)

Rules for Classification

There should be histological confirmation of the disease to permit division of cases by histological type.

The following are the procedures for assessment of the T, N and M categories:

T categories   Physical examination
N categories   Physical examination
M categories   Physical examination and imaging

Regional Lymph Nodes

The regional lymph nodes are the preauricular, submandibular and cervical lymph nodes.

TNM Clinical Classification

T – Primary Tumour

TX   Primary tumour cannot be assessed
T0   No evidence of primary tumour

T1   Tumour 2.5 cm or less in greatest dimension, limited to the lacrimal gland

T2   Tumour 2.5 cm or less in greatest dimension, invading the periosteum of the fossa of the lacrimal gland

T3   Tumour more than 2.5 cm but not more than 5 cm in greatest dimension
  T3 a   Tumour limited to the lacrimal gland

T3b   Tumour invades the periosteum of the fossa of the
      lacrimal gland
T4   Tumour invades 5 cm in greatest dimension
T4a   Tumour invades orbital soft tissues, optic nerve, or
      globe, but *without* bone invasion
T4b   Tumour invades orbital soft tissues, optic nerve, or
      globe, *with* bone invasion

N - Regional Lymph Nodes

See definitions p.146.

M - Distant Metastasis

See definitions p.146.

pTNM Pathological Classification

The pT, pN and pM categories correspond to the T, N and M
categories.

G Histopathological Grading

GX   Grade of differentiation cannot assessed
G1   Well differentiated
G2   Moderately differentiated; includes adenoid cystic carci-
     noma without basaloid (solid) pattern
G3   Poorly differentiated; includes adenoid cystic carcinoma
     with basaloid (solid) pattern
G4   Undifferentiated

Stage Grouping

No stage grouping is at present recommended.

Summary

Lacrimal Gland Carcinoma		
T1		$\leqslant$ 2.5 cm, limited to gland
T2		$\leqslant$ 2.5 cm, periosteum
T3		> 2.5 cm to 5 cm
	T3a	Limited to gland
	T3b	Periosteum
T4		> 5 cm
	T4a	Orbit but not orbital bone
	T4b	Orbit and orbital bone
N1		Regional

BRAIN TUMOURS (ICD-O 191)

Rules for Classification

The classification applies to all brain tumours. There should be histological confirmation of the disease. An N/pN classification does not apply to brain tumours.

The following are the procedures for assessment of T and M categories:

T categories   Physical examination and imaging
M categories   Physical examination and imaging

TM Clinical Classification

T – Primary Tumour

TX   Primary tumour cannot be assessed
T0   No evidence of primary tumour

Supratentorial Tumours

T1   Tumour 5 cm or less in greatest dimension, limited to one side
T2   Tumour more than 5 cm in greatest dimension, limited to one side
T3   Tumour invades or encroaches upon the ventricular system
T4   Tumour crosses the midline of the brain, invades the opposite hemisphere, or invades infratentorially

Infratentorial Tumours

T1   Tumour 3 cm or less in greatest dimension, limited to one
      side
T2   Tumour more than 3 cm in greatest dimension, limited to
      one side
T3   Tumour invades or encroaches upon the ventricular system
T4   Tumour crosses the midline of the brain, invades the oppo-
      site hemisphere, or invades supratentorially

M – Distant Metastasis

MX   Presence of distant metastasis cannot be assessed
M0   No distant metastasis
M1   Distant metastasis

pTM Pathological Classification

The pT and pM categories correspond to the T and M categories.

G Histopathological Grading

GX   Grade cannot be assessed
G1   Well differentiated
G2   Moderately differentiated
G3   Poorly differentiated
G4   Undifferentiated

R Classification

The absence or presence of residual tumour after treatment may be described by the symbol R:

RX Presence of residual tumour cannot be assessed
R0 No residual tumour
R1 Microscopic tumour
R2 Macroscopic residual tumour

Stage Grouping

Stage I A	G1	T1	M0
Stage I B	G1	T2, T3	M0
Stage II A	G2	T1	M0
Stage II B	G2	T2, T3	M0
Stage III A	G3	T1	M0
Stage III B	G3	T2, T3	M0
Stage IV	G1	T4	M0
	G2	T4	M0
	G3	T4	M0
	G4	Any T	M0
	Any G	Any T	M1

Summary

Brain	
	Supratentorial
T1	One side, ≤ 5 cm
T2	One side > 5 cm
T3	Ventricular system
T4	Opposite side, infratentorial
	Infratentorial
T1	One side, ≤ 3 cm
T2	One side, > 3 cm
T3	Ventricular system
T4	Opposite side, supratentorial
	All Sites
G1	Well differentiated
G2	Moderately differentiated
G3	Poorly differentiated
G4	Undifferentiated

HODGKIN'S DISEASE

Introductory Notes

At the present time it is not considered practical to propose a TNM classification for Hodgkin's disease.

Following the development of the Ann Arbor classification for Hodgkin's disease in 1971 the significance of two important observations with major impact on staging has been appreciated. First, extralymphatic disease, if localized and related to adjacent lymph node disease, does not adversely affect the survival of patients. Secondly, laparotomy with splenectomy has been introduced as a method of obtaining more information on the extent of the disease within the abdomen.

A stage classification based on information from histopathological examination of the spleen and lymph nodes obtained at laparotomy cannot be compared with another done without such exploration. Therefore two systems of classification are presented, a clinical (cS) and a pathological (pS).

Clinical Staging (cS)

Although recognized as incomplete, this is easily performed and should be reproducible from one centre to another. It is determined by history, clinical examination, imaging, blood analysis and the initial biopsy report. Bone marrow biopsy must be taken from a clinically or radiologically non-involved area of bone.

Liver Involvement. Clinical evidence of liver involvement must include either enlargement of the liver and at least an abnormal serum alkaline phosphatase level and two different liver function test abnormalities, or an abnormal liver demonstrated by imaging and one abnormal liver function test.

Spleen Involvement. Clinical evidence of spleen involvement is accepted if there is palpable enlargement of the spleen confirmed by imaging.

Lymphatic and Extralymphatic Disease. The lymphatic structures are as follows:

Lymph nodes	Waldeyer's ring
Spleen	Appendix
Thymus	Peyer's patches

   The lymph nodes are grouped into regions and one or more (2, 3 etc.) may be involved. The spleen is designated S and extralymphatic organs or sites E.

   Lung involvement limited to one lobe, or perihilar extension associated with ipsilateral lymphadenopathy, or unilateral pleural effusion with or without lung involvement but with hilar lymphadenopathy, are considered as *localized* extralymphatic diseases.

   Liver involvement is always considered as *diffuse* extralymphatic disease.

Pathological Staging (pS)

This takes into account additional data and has a higher degree of precision. It should be applied whenever possible. The various categories should be subscripted − (minus) or + (plus) according to the results of histopathological examination.

Histopathological Information

This is classified by symbols indicating the tissue sampled. The following notation is common to the distant metastases (or M1 categories) of all regions classified by the TNM system. However, in order to conform with the Ann Arbor classification, the initial letters used in that system are also given.

Pulmonay	PUL or L	Bone marrow	MAR or M
Osseous	OSS or O	Pleura	PLE or P
Hepatic	HEP or H	Peritoneum	PER
Brain	BRA	Skin	SKI or D
Lymph nodes	LYM or N	Other	OTH

Additional Descriptors

When appropriate, the y symbol, the r symbol and the C-factor category may be added (see p. 9).

Clinical Stages (cS)

Stage I   Involvement of a single lymph node region (I), or localized involvement of a single extralymphatic organ or site (I_E)

Stage II   Involvement of two or more lymph node regions on the same side of the diaphragm (II), or localized involvement of a single extralymphatic organ or site and its regional lymph node(s) with or without involvement of other lymph node regions on the same side of the diaphragm (II_E)

Note: The number of lymph note regions involved may be indicated by a subscript (e.g. II_3)

Stage III   Involvement of lymph node regions on both sides of the diaphragm (III), which may also be accompanied by localized involvement of an associated extralymphatic organ or site (III_E), or by involvement of the spleen (III_S), or both (III_{E+S})

Stage IV   Disseminated (multifocal) involvement of one or more extralymphatic organs, with or without associated lymph node involvement; or isolated extralymphatic organ involvement with distant (non-regional) nodal involvement.

Note: The site of Stage IV disease is identified further by specifying sites according to the notations listed on p. 177.

Symptoms A and B

Each stage should be divided into A and B according to the absence or presence of defined general symptoms. These are:
1. Unexplained weight loss of more than 10% of the usual body weight in the 6 months prior to first attendance
2. Unexplained fever with temperature above 38 °C
3. Night sweats

Note: Pruritus alone does not qualify for B classification nor does a short, febrile illness associated with a known infection.

Pathological Stages (pS)

The definitions of the four stages follow the same criteria as the clinical stages but with the additional information obtained following laparotomy. Splenectomy, liver biopsy, lymph node biopsy and marrow biopsy are mandatory for the establishment of pathological stages. The results of these biopsies are recorded as indicated above (see p. 176 and 177).

Summary

Stage	Hodgkin's Disease	Substage
Stage I	Single node region Localized single extralymphatic organ/site	I_E
Stage II	Two or more node regions, same side of diaphragm Localized single extralymphatic organ/site with its regional nodes, $\pm$ other node regions same side of diaphragm	II_E
Stage III	Node regions both sides of diaphragm $\pm$ Localized single extralymphatic organ/site spleen both	III_E III_S III_{E+S}
Stage IV	Diffuse involvement extralymphatic organ(s) $\pm$ regional Isolated extralymphatic organ and non-regional nodes	
All stages divided	Without weight loss/fever/sweats With weight loss/fever/sweats	A B

NON-HODGKIN'S LYMPHOMA

As in Hodgkin's disease, at the present time it is not considered practical to propose a TNM classification for Non-Hodgkin's lymphoma. Since no other convincing and tested staging system is available, the Ann Arbor classification is recommended with the same modification as for Hodgkin's disease (see p. 175).

PAEDIATRIC TUMOURS

Introductory Notes

The tumours classified are nephroblastoma, neuroblastoma and soft tissue sarcomas of childhood. These tumours are classified according to the recommendations of the Société Internationale d'Oncologie Pédiatrique (SIOP). They have the approval of UICC and the national TNM committees including AJCC.

The rules for the classification of paediatric tumours differ in one respect from those applicable to other sites. It is necessary to include a category for those cases in which a surgical exploration is done and in which a non-resectable tumour is found. Such cases are designated pT3c or, if following previous non-surgical treatment, ypT3c.

Each tumour type is described under the following headings:

Rules for classification with the procedures for assessing the T, N and M categories. Additional methods may be used when they enhance the accuracy of appraisal before treatment
Anatomical regions where appropriate
Definition of the regional lymph nodes
TNM Clinical classification
pTNM Pathological classification
Stage grouping
Summary

Additional Descriptors

When appropriate, the y symbol, the r symbol and the C-factor category may be added to the classification (see p. 9).

Distant Metastasis

The definitions of the M categories for all paediatric tumours are:

M – Distant Metastasis

MX   Presence of distant metastasis cannot be assessed
M0   No distant metastasis
M1   Distant metastasis

For all regions the categories M1 and pM1 may be further specified according to the following notation:

Pulmonary	PUL	Bone marrow	MAR
Osseous	OSS	Pleura	PLE
Hepatic	HEP	Peritoneum	PER
Brain	BRA	Skin	SKI
Lymph nodes	LYM	Other	OTH

Nephroblastoma (Wilms' Tumour)
(ICD-O 189.0)

Rules for Classification

There should be histological confirmation of the disease.

The following are the procedures for assessment of the T, N and M categories. Additional methods may be used when they enhance the accuracy of appraisal before treatment.

T categories	Physical examination and urography; any other diagnostic technique may be employed before treatment
N categories	Physical examination and imaging (Note: The assessment of N categories is not considered relevant)
M categories	Physical examination and imaging

Regional Lymph Nodes

The regional lymph nodes are the hilar, para-aortic and para-caval nodes between the diaphragm and the bifurcation of the aorta. Other involved lymph nodes are considered distant metastases.

TNM Clinical Classification

T – Primary Tumour

TX   Primary tumour cannot be assessed
T0   No evidence of primary tumour

T1   Unilateral tumour 80 cm^2 or less in area (including kidney)[1]

T2   Unilateral tumour more than 80 cm^2 in area (including kidney)

Note: [1] The area is calculated by multiplying the vertical and horizontal dimensions of the radiological shadow of the tumour and kidney ($a \times b$).

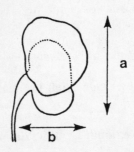

T3   Unilateral tumour rupture before treatment
T4   Bilateral tumours

N – Regional Lymph Nodes

NX   Regional lymph nodes cannot be assessed
N0   No regional lymph node metastasis
N1   Regional lymph node metastasis

M – Distant Metastasis

See definitions p. 182.

pTNM Pathological Classification

pT – Primary Tumour

pTX Primary tumour cannot be assessed
pT0 No evidence of primary tumour

pT1 Intrarenal tumour completely encapsulated, excision complete and margins histologically free

pT2 Tumour invades beyond the capsule or renal parenchyma[2], excision complete

pT3 Tumour invades beyond the capsule or renal parenchyma[2], excision incomplete *or* pre-operative or operative rupture

    pT3a Microscopic residual tumour limited to tumour bed

    pT3b Macroscopic residual tumour or spillage or malignant ascites

    pT3c Surgical exploration, tumour not resected

pT4 Bilateral tumours

Note: [2] This includes breach of the renal capsule and/or tumour seen microscopically outside the capsule; tumour adhesions microscopically confirmed, infiltrations of, or tumour thrombus within, the renal vessels outside the kidney; infiltration of the renal pelvis and/or ureter, peri-pelvic and pericalyceal fat.

pN – Regional Lymph Nodes

pNX Regional lymph nodes cannot be assessed
pN0 No regional lymph node metastasis

pN1 Regional lymph node metastasis

    pN1a Regional lymph node metastasis completely resected

    pN1b Regional lymph node metastasis incompletely resected

pM – Distant Metastasis

The pM categories correspond to the M categories.

Clinical Stage Grouping (TNM, cTNM)

Stage I	T1	N0	M0
Stage II	T2	N0	M0
Stage III	T1	N1	M0
	T2	N1	M0
	T3	Any N	M0
Stage IV A	T1	Any N	M1
	T2	Any N	M1
	T3	Any N	M1
Stage IV B	T4	Any N	Any M

Pathological Stage Grouping (pTNM)

Stage I	pT1	pN0	pM0
Stage II	pT1	pN1a	pM0
	pT2	pN0, pN1a	pM0
Stage III A	pT3a	pN0, pN1a	pM0
Stage III B	pT1	pN1b	pM0
	pT2	pN1b	pM0
	pT3a	pN1b	pM0
	pT3b	Any pN	pM0
	pT3c	Any pN	pM0
Stage IV A	pT1	Any pN	pM1
	pT2	Any pN	pM1
	pT3a	Any pN	pM1
	pT3b	Any pN	pM1
	pT3c	Any pN	pM1
Stage IV B	pT4	Any pN	Any pM

Summary

TNM	Nephroblastoma		pTNM
T1	Tumour $\leqslant 80$ cm^2	Encapsulated, excision complete	pT1
T2	Tumour > 80 cm^2	With invasion, excision complete	pT2
T3	Rupture before treatment	Excision incomplete, microscopic residual tumour	pT3a
		Excision incomplete, macroscopic residual tumour	pT3b
		Tumour not resected	pT3c
T4	Bilateral tumours	Bilateral tumours	pT4
N1	Regional	Metastasis completely resected	pN1a
		Metastasis incompletely resected	pN1b

Neuroblastoma

The same principles apply to ganglioneuroblastoma.

Rules for Classification

There should be histological confirmation of the disease and/or confirmation by biochemical tests.

The following are the procedures for assessment of the T, N and M categories. Additional methods may be used when they enhance the accuracy of appraisal before treatment.

T categories	Physical examination, imaging including intravenous urography and chest X-ray
N categories	Physical examination and imaging
M categories	Physical examination and imaging including skeletal survey and bone marrow examination

Anatomical Regions

The primary tumour site should be indicated according to the following notation:

Cervical	CER	Pelvic	PEL
Thoracic	THO	Other	OTH
Abdominal	ABD		

Note: Dumbbell tumours should be indentified by the prefix D.

Regional Lymph Nodes

The regional lymph nodes are as follows:

Cervical region   Cervical and supraclavicular nodes
Thoracic region   Intrathoracic and infraclavicular nodes
Abdominal and   Subdiaphragmatic, intraabdominal and pel-
pelvic regions   vic nodes, including the external iliac nodes
Other regions   The appropriate regional lymph nodes

TNM Clinical Classification

T – Primary Tumour

Because it is often impossible to differentiate between the primary tumour and the adjacent lymph nodes, the T assessment relates to the total mass. When there is doubt between multicentricity and metastasis, the latter is presumed.

Note: Size is estimated clinically and/or radiologically. For classification the larger measurement should be used.

TX   Primary tumour cannot be assessed
T0   No evidence of primary tumour

T1   Single tumour 5 cm or less in greatest dimension
T2   Single tumour more than 5 cm but not more than 10 cm in greatest dimension
T3   Single tumour more than 10 cm in greatest dimension
T4   Multicentric tumours occurring simultaneously

N – Regional Lymph Nodes

NX   Regional lymph nodes cannot be assessed
N0   No regional lymph node metastasis
N1   Regional lymph node metastasis

M – Distant Metastasis

See definitions p. 182.

pTNM Pathological Classification

pT – Primary Tumour

pTX   Primary tumour cannot be assessed
pT0   No evidence of primary tumour

pT1   Excision of tumour complete and margins histologically
        free
pT2   The category does not apply to neuroblastoma
pT3   Residual tumour
        pT3a   Microscopic residual tumour
        pT3b   Macroscopic residual tumour or grossly incom-
                plete excision
        pT3c   Surgical exploration, tumour not resected
pT4   Multicentric tumour

pN – Regional Lymph Nodes

pNX   Regional lymph nodes cannot be assessed
pN0   No regional lymph node metastasis
pN1   Regional lymph node metastasis
        pN1a   Regional lymph node metastasis completely
                resected
        pN1b   Regional lymph node metastasis incompletely
                resected

pM – Distant Metastasis

The pM categories correspond to the M categories.

Clinical Stage Grouping (TNM, cTNM)

Stage I	T1	N0	M0
Stage II	T2	N0	M0
Stage III	T1	N1	M0
	T2	N1	M0
	T3	Any N	M0
Stage IV A	T1	Any N	M1
	T2	Any N	M1
	T3	Any N	M1
Stage IV B	T4	Any N	Any M

Pathological Stage Grouping (pTNM)

Stage I	pT1	pN0	pM0
Stage II	pT1	pN1 a	pM0
Stage III A	pT3 a	pN0, pN1 a	pM0
Stage III B	pT1	pN1 b	pM0
	pT3 a	pN1 b	pM0
	pT3 b	Any pN	pM0
	pT3 c	Any pN	pM0
Stage IV A	pT1	Any pN	pM1
	pT3 a	Any pN	pM1
	pT3 b	Any pN	pM1
	pT3 c	Any pN	pM1
Stage IV B	pT4	Any pN	Any pM

Summary

TNM	Neuroblastoma		*pTNM*
T1	Tumour ⩽ 5 cm	Excision complete	pT1
T2	Tumour > 5 to 10 cm	(Not applicable)	pT2
T3	Tumour > 10 cm	Microscopic residual tumour	pT3a
		Macroscopic residual tumour	pT3b
		Non-resectable tumour	pT3c
T4	Multicentric tumour	Multicentric tumour	pT4
N1	Regional	Metastasis completely resected	pN1a
		Metastasis incompletely resected	pN1b

Soft Tissue Sarcomas – Paediatric

Rules for Classification

The classification is designed to apply particularly to rhabdo-myosarcoma in childhood (ICD-O M 8900/3) but may be used for other soft tissue sarcomas in childhood (listed on p. 80). There should be histological confirmation of the disease.

The following are the procedures for assessment of the T, N and M categories. Additional methods may be used when they enhance the accuracy of appraisal before treatment.

T categories	Physical examination and imaging appropriate to the anatomical region
N categories	Physical examination and relevant imaging
M categories	Physical examination and imaging; in rhabdo-myosarcoma bone marrow examination is recommended

Anatomical Regions

The primary tumour site should be indicated according to the following notation:

Orbit	ORB	Abdomen (including walls and viscera)	ABD
Head and neck	HEA		
Limbs	LIM	Thorax (including walls, diaphragm and viscera)	THO
Pelvis (including walls, genital tract and viscera)	PEL	Other	OTH

Regional Lymph Nodes

The regional lymph nodes are those appropriate to the situation of the primary tumour, for example:

Head and neck	Cervical and supraclavicular lymph nodes
Abdominal and pelvic	Subdiaphragmatic, intra-abdominal and ilio-inguinal lymph nodes
Upper limbs	Ipsilateral epitrochlear and axillary lymph nodes
Lower limbs	Ipsilateral popliteal and inguinal lymph nodes

In the case of unilateral tumours, all contralateral involved lymph nodes are considered to be distant metastasis.

TNM Clinical Classification

T – Primary Tumour

TX   Primary tumour cannot be assessed
T0   No evidence of primary tumour

T1   Tumour limited to organ or tissue of origin
       T1a   Tumour 5 cm or less in greatest dimension
       T1b   Tumour more than 5 cm in greatest dimension
T2   Tumour invades contiguous organ(s) or tissue(s) and/or with adjacent malignant effusion
       T2a   Tumour 5 cm or less in greatest dimension
       T2b   Tumour more than 5 cm in greatest dimension

Note: The categories T3 and T4 do not apply. The existence of more than one tumour is generally considered a primary tumour with distant metastasis.

N – Regional Lymph Nodes

NX   Regional lymph nodes cannot be assessed
N0   No regional lymph node metastasis
N1   Regional lymph node metastasis

M – Distant Metastasis

See definitions p. 182

pTNM Pathological Classification

pT – Primary Tumour

pTX   Primary tumour cannot be assessed
pT0   No evidence of primary tumour

pT1   Tumour limited to organ or tissue of origin; excision complete and margins histologically free

pT2   Tumour invades beyond the organ or tissue of origin; excision complete and margins histologically free

pT3   Tumour invades beyond the organ or tissue of origin; excision incomplete

     pT3a   Microscopic residual tumour
     pT3b   Macroscopic residual tumour or adjacent malignant effusion
     pT3c   Surgical exploration, tumour not resected

pN – Regional Lymph Nodes

pNX   Regional lymph nodes cannot be assessed
pN0   No regional lymph node metastasis
pN1   Regional lymph node metastasis

     pN1a   Regional lymph node metastasis completely resected
     pN1b   Regional lymph node metastasis incompletely resected

pM – Distant Metastasis

The pM categories correspond to the M categories.

Clinical Stage Grouping (TNM, cTNM)

Stage I	T1a	N0	M0
	T1b	N0	M0
Stage II	T2a	N0	M0
	T2b	N0	M0
Stage III	Any T	N1	M0
Stage IV	Any T	Any N	M1

Pathological Stage Grouping (pTNM)

Stage I	pT1	pN0	pM0
Stage II	pT1	pN1a	pM0
	pT2	pN0, pN1a	pM0
Stage III A	pT3a	pN0, pN1a	pM0
Stage III B	pT3b	Any pN	pM0
	pT3c	Any pN	pM0
	Any pT	pN1b	pM0
Stage IV	Any pT	Any pN	pM1

Summary

TNM	Soft Tissue Sarcoma – Paediatric		*pTNM*
T1	Limited to organ/tissue	Limited to organ, excision complete	pT1
T1a	≤5 cm		
T1b	>5cm		
T2	Invades contiguous organs/tissues	Invades beyond organ, excision complete	pT2
T2a	≤5 cm		
T2b	>5 cm		

TNM	Soft Tissue Sarcoma – Paediatric		*pTNM*
T3/4	(Not applicable)	Excision incomplete	pT3
		Microscopic residual tumour	pT3a
		Macroscopic residual tumour	pT3b
		Tumour not resected	pT3c
N1	Regional	Metastasis completely resected	pN1a
		Metastasis incompletely resected	pN1b